Stoned

CURRENT

Stoned

A Doctor's Case for Medical Marijuana

David Casarett, M.D.

CURRENT

CURRENT

An imprint of Penguin Random House LLC
375 Hudson Street
New York, New York 10014

ISBN 978-1-59184-767-0

Printed in the United States of America
1   3   5   7   9   10   8   6   4   2

Set in Minion Pro Regular and Chalet Nineteen Sixty
Designed by Amy Hill

For Caleb.
I hope that he found the relief he was searching for.

What is a weed?
A plant whose virtues
have never been discovered.

—RALPH WALDO EMERSON[1]

Contents

Stoned

1

The Blacksmith and the Boxer

The mobile home has traveled many hard miles. Like old luggage, its tan exterior is scuffed and faded and marred by countless dents. In the gusty wind blowing across the surrounding field on the outskirts of Denver, its frame rocks restlessly on bald tires, making it seem alive. The windows are obscured by curtains. A poster on the door shows the outline of a human-shaped shooting target, pocked with bullet holes. The caption below it reads "There's nothing in here worth dying for."

I turn to the man standing next to me. Nathan Pollack is in his seventies, with snow-white hair and a whorled white beard that ends in a sharp point at his chin. His black beret and rumpled tweed sport coat make him look like he could be a professor at a small liberal arts college. He is in fact a hospice doctor, like me, and he's about to introduce me to a patient whose story I very much want to hear.

I knock, and the door opens a few inches, revealing the head of an enormous dog with bulbous eyes and small, clipped ears. His intimidation potential is elevated a bit by the fact that his teeth are at the level of my throat.

It turns out that the dog—all eighty pounds of him—just wants someone to scratch behind his ears. Still, I let Pollack go in first.

Inside, the mobile home smells of stale marijuana smoke, dog, old socks, and compost. The interior is dark despite the bright winter day outside. Several heavy quilts cover the windows as insulation against the biting wind, and another covers the doorway that leads to the cab in front. The cozy womblike space is crammed with a bed, two small chairs, and a tiny kitchen area. There's faded wallpaper and a mock-Tudor ceiling constructed of stucco interspersed with faux wood beams. It's oddly homey.

As my eyes adjust to the dark, I get a good look at the man Pollack has brought me to meet. Caleb* is in his forties, lean and wiry. His neatly trimmed mustache is at odds with brown hair that's long and boyishly unkempt. He's sitting cross-legged on his bed, warmly dressed in a thermal long-sleeved shirt, a flannel shirt, jeans, and well-worn athletic socks.

Caleb's hands are shaking, and I recognize the resting tremor of Parkinson's disease. He tells me that he got that diagnosis several years ago and thinks the unusually early onset is probably a result of his work as a blacksmith and a welder. "You inhale every heavy metal known to man," he says. "No surprise that they do all kinds of damage to your brain."

I ask him his dog's name, and Caleb's face contorts into what might pass for a smile.

"Rocky."

Of course. What else would you call a boxer? I laugh, and Caleb does, too. He clutches his left side in obvious pain. Then that passes, and he starts to tell me the story I came to hear.

Two years ago, he was diagnosed with rectal cancer. He received what he described as "aggressive" treatment in Wisconsin. "Some days I didn't think I could take any more," he says. "But then I'd go by the children's hospital and I'd watch those kids playing outside and I'd think, 'If they can handle this, then I can, too.'"

---

* "Caleb" isn't his real name. Here and throughout, I've used first-name pseudonyms for all of the patients I've met, as well as for anyone else who might get into legal trouble for their marijuana-related activities. The people for whom I've included full (real) names gave me their permission to do so and spoke on the record.

His doctors told him that treatment could prolong his life, but wouldn't cure him. So he suffered through as much treatment as he could stand, and then he drove west to Colorado where he knew he'd be able to get marijuana legally to treat his pain and control his nausea.

Along the way, he also discovered that marijuana didn't only relieve those symptoms.

"It also keeps me from being an asshole." He pauses. "Well, too much of an asshole, anyway. It sort of blunts the sharp edges. I'm not so pissed off all the time about everything—at everyone."

"Having cancer sucks," he admits. "But when you've got your red card"—that's Colorado's medical marijuana card—"dying sucks a little less."

It turned out, however, that getting marijuana wasn't so easy.

As soon as he parked his mobile home in this suburb outside of Denver, Caleb found Pollack's hospice, which promised free marijuana to its patients. That's essential, because Caleb lives on about $600 a month. But Pollack's hospice had stopped providing marijuana because the management didn't want to run afoul of federal laws that still classify marijuana as an illegal substance. So once he was in Denver, Caleb wasn't able to get marijuana from Pollack's hospice, and he couldn't afford to buy his own.

As Caleb tells his story, he drops the courtly politeness with which he'd greeted me a few minutes ago, and his language becomes increasingly laced with profanity. He goes on to say how much he depends on the marijuana he smokes. But he can't afford it.

"Oh, there's plenty of places to buy. That's the hell of it. Sure it's legal, but . . ." He rubs his thumb and forefinger together in the universal sign for money. "You have to be able to pay."

I ask him if he'd found another hospice that could give him marijuana, and he grins.

"No, I didn't really look." He winks at Pollack. "I'll complain, sure. I'm not shy. Especially when I'm pissed off. But these are good folks. They take good care of me."

He's stayed with Pollack's hospice, and he's gotten marijuana from so-called angels in the community who make donations directly to him. That keeps the hospice out of trouble, which is fine with Caleb.

"I wouldn't want anybody going to jail for me."

Besides, he has a plan.

"I'm growing my own. See?" He points.

To my left, at the rear of the mobile home, there's a grow light suspended over a plastic tub. The light sways gently in the wind, casting undulating shadows of what looks like about thirty immature marijuana plants. A few are about eighteen inches tall and look like they might start budding in a couple of weeks. But most are no more than a couple of inches high.

Caleb admits that those smaller plants were the result of an accident. Literally. He went to pick up plants from someone who was moving and wanted to give them a good home. But problems ensued.

"I'm not the best driver, you know?"

I look back at the psychoactive garden. I nod.

Caleb is a little vague about details, but apparently while he was driving, the microwave fell off its shelf and several plants lost their lives. He salvaged what he could by taking cuttings and creating clones, which are the Lilliputian plants that take up most of his little greenhouse.

I notice a box on a shelf behind him. It's labeled COMFORT KIT.

This is a set of medications that many hospices provide to their patients in case of emergencies. It generally includes morphine for pain, and benzodiazepines like Valium for anxiety and seizures.

Has he used them?

"Hell no. They don't work. Why would I waste my time with them?" He gestures at a dime bag of marijuana on the kitchen counter. "That's all I need, right there."

Caleb recognizes the irony of this arrangement. His hospice can provide a variety of drugs such as morphine free of charge. These are drugs that have the potential to cause a fatal overdose, and which can be addictive. But the drug that really helps him—marijuana—is out of reach.

"Those are your tax dollars at work, man. You're paying for the government to spend money on that box of shitty drugs that I'm not going to touch. That's a waste. But what I really need, they can't give me. Does that make sense?"

I admit that it doesn't. As if in agreement, Rocky the boxer hops off the bed where he'd been sitting with Caleb and rests his chin on my leg.

Does Medical Marijuana "Work"?

In Pollack's Toyota, heading back to Denver, I think about Caleb's predicament. I'm a little shell-shocked by what I've heard. I'd always thought of medical marijuana as a joke. Or a "treatment" that would always be described in just that way, hemmed in by ironic quotes.

Yet Caleb is dying and in pain. And he wants it—needs it—for relief. This isn't a guy who wants to get high for fun. This is a man who has led a hard life and who doesn't want to suffer more than he has to.

Some patients I've taken care of in my work as a hospice and palliative care doctor have admitted to me that they use marijuana for symptoms like pain or nausea. (And I'm pretty sure that for every patient who has been honest with me about using marijuana, there are many more who haven't.) They've made it into a joke, just as I have.

Laughing uncomfortably, one Vietnam veteran told me he started smoking half a joint per day more than twenty years ago to control his PTSD symptoms. Better to be high than out of his head, right? I laughed, too, and we moved on to talk about his cancer pain that I was treating.

I'm pretty sure I shouldn't have laughed. Like Caleb, that veteran needed help. He'd found something that relieved his symptoms, and he needed my support.

I don't remember what I said. Probably some version of what all doctors say when confronted with alternative medicine we don't understand (or, in the case of marijuana, common but usually illegal). "Well, I guess it can't hurt." Or, "If it makes you feel better . . ." But I didn't ask him whether it helped him, or how.

Marijuana is the *only* thing that's helped Caleb. This is a guy who is letting $100 worth of morphine and other interesting drugs sit in his closet. He'd rather have a joint.

What's more, Caleb turned to marijuana to avoid drugs like morphine. Not only is he convinced that marijuana is helpful, he's convinced that it's better than the legal drugs he can get for free. It might be safer, too.

Does marijuana "work"?

When I met Caleb in early 2014, the debate about legalizing medical marijuana was just beginning to get national attention. But that debate was about ethics and morality. Do people have a right to use it? And how should laws be crafted?

No one was really talking seriously about whether marijuana has any medical value. Or whether it's safe. Or, setting the bar a little lower, whether it's at least as safe as other drugs that doctors prescribe.

My goal with this book is to shift the national discussion, and to bring these questions about effectiveness and safety to the forefront. These are the questions we really need to be asking. And these are the questions that I wanted to be able to answer in order to decide, as a physician, what advice I should give my patients when they ask me whether they should use medical marijuana.

In this book I've attempted to look carefully—and critically—at the evidence. I searched for high-quality published studies, and I interviewed researchers who are doing those studies. In short, I subjected medical marijuana to the same scrutiny that I'd give to the drugs that the pharmaceutical industry tries to sell to physicians like me.

First, I investigated whether marijuana works as medicine. I scoured medical journals, interviewed patients, and visited physicians and researchers. I wanted to find out what we know about marijuana's effect on conditions related to the brain, such as insomnia and PTSD and seizures. I wanted to learn whether it could be useful in treating physical symptoms such as nausea and weight loss, and whether the ingredients in marijuana might actually treat diseases like dementia, multiple sclerosis, or cancer.

Then I explored how people get marijuana into their systems. That might seem like a silly question, but it's not an easy one to answer. I learned how to infuse the ingredients of marijuana into beer and wine and brownies and ointment. I discovered how effective joints and bongs are at delivering marijuana's ingredients to our brains compared to newer technologies such as vaporizers. Along the way, I learned how to make hash. I even discovered what I've been told is the world's best pot brownie recipe. (It's on page 261, in case you want to skip ahead.)

All that is great, but is marijuana *safe*? For most readers of this book, this might be the most important question. So I sifted through the evidence about whether long-term use causes brain damage, or mental illness, or addiction. I discovered there are other risks of marijuana use beyond its effects on the brain—from infertility to shrinking penises and everything in between. I'll also share my own misguided experiences with medical marijuana, and I'll take you for a drive with one of my patients shortly after he smoked a joint.

Next, how are patients like Caleb figuring out whether marijuana could help them? How do they sort through the risks and potential benefits of this stuff? Where do they turn for advice? And how reliable is that advice?

Finally, what does the future hold for medical marijuana? Is it on its way to being the next superdrug? Should it be legalized and made more available? Or is this all merely hype to justify recreational drug use?

These are high-stakes questions. As of this writing, twenty-three states and the District of Columbia have legalized marijuana for medical purposes, and a few have allowed it for recreational purposes, too. It seems very likely that medical marijuana will be legal in most states in the not-too-distant future. And in states where it's legal, lots of people are using it. According to one study in California, 5 percent of people surveyed had used medical marijuana.[1] That means that my questions about marijuana's effectiveness, and especially its safety, have big implications for hundreds of thousands of people.

These numbers are likely to increase further as more dispensaries open to sell marijuana. That was the conclusion of another study in

California that surveyed more than eight thousand people in fifty cities and mapped their proximity to marijuana dispensaries. The results: people who were close to a dispensary used more marijuana.[2]

The states that have legalized it have done so with very broad criteria. You can use it for chronic pain, anxiety, insomnia, arthritis, and a wide variety of other conditions. Most people who are embracing it are not near the end of life. They are students, construction workers, police officers, teachers, and—I can attest—at least one doctor.

If medical marijuana works, then its growing popularity is good news. But if it doesn't work, then it's an enormous waste of time and money. Even worse, if marijuana isn't safe, we'll have an enormous public health crisis on our hands. As you'll see later in the book, if lots of people are using medical marijuana, even a very small risk could result in lots of people being harmed or even killed.

As I started writing this book, the public was just beginning to recognize those risks. For instance, one study found that long-term marijuana use was associated with brain atrophy—in other words, brain shrinkage.[3] But shortly after that rather alarming study made headlines, *The New York Times* published an editorial in favor of legalizing medical marijuana, and discounting its risks. So is it safe or not?[4]

Whether marijuana is safe and effective is particularly important because its safety will determine how it's regulated. For much of its recent history, marijuana has been classified in the United States as a Schedule I substance. This category is reserved for drugs like heroin that are believed to have significant risks but no known medical benefits. As long as marijuana continues to live in that category, it's going to be impossible to create national rules about how it can be used, prescribed, and distributed. It's also very difficult for researchers to do studies that can help us figure out whether and how it works. And patients like Caleb won't be able to get it from a hospice.

I wasn't sure where I'd come out on the other end of this journey. Pro or con? I'm also not sure which side you'll be on when you reach the last chapter. But no matter what your verdict, I think I can promise you an interesting journey that will give you enough information to make up your own mind about whether marijuana could help you.

Finally, a book about pot wouldn't be complete without some caveats.

First, a word about names: Throughout this book, I'll be referring to "marijuana," over the objections of some purists who prefer the term *cannabis*, as in *Cannabis sativa*. They correctly note that the name *marijuana* (actually *marihuana*, imported from Mexico) was bestowed by narcotics enforcement officials back in the 1940s as a way to scare off potential users. Back then, the connotations of foreignness and crime (think *Reefer Madness*) were enough to deter a few people. (Of course, those connotations also probably made the stuff irresistible to others.) Although I admit that cannabis is the proper term, marijuana is so widely recognized that I've chosen to use this name instead, with all due apologies to terminological purists.

Second, you shouldn't rely on this book as your sole source of medical advice. If you want to learn how to treat symptoms like pain, you should also see a physician.

However, this book will help you decide whether medical marijuana might help you. I've written it for people like my own patients, and like Caleb, who are struggling with distressing symptoms and looking for help. It's intended to be a summary of the sort of advice I would want them to have when they're deciding whether medical marijuana might help them.

For instance, I'll tell you how medical marijuana can be helpful, and what symptoms it's most effective in treating. I'll also warn you about marijuana's risks, and how you can avoid them. Along the way, I'll tell you enough about the science of medical marijuana to understand how it works, and what it might be able to do for us in the future.

2

The Girl Who Talked to Cats: Marijuana's Benefits for the Brain

The woman sitting in the seat next to me in the waiting room of this medical marijuana clinic is in her early thirties, blond, and very attractive. Julie is dressed in the sort of fleece-and-spandex garb that might signal a recent Ashtanga yoga session, or an impending hundred-mile ultramarathon. She is undoubtedly very healthy, and could, in a fit of poetic license, be described as "glowing."

Like the other people sitting around us, she has come to this Denver clinic to get a card that will let her purchase marijuana legally to treat a variety of symptoms and conditions. Unlike everyone around us, though, she doesn't appear to have any such problems. In fact, Julie seems about as healthy as it's possible for any human being to be.

That's why I struck up a conversation with her, and that's why she's telling me about how marijuana has changed her life.

"It's totally reset my brain," she tells me earnestly.

Julie explains that smoking a joint every day—and sometimes more—has given her a calmer outlook. She sleeps better and has more energy during the day. Marijuana has reduced her anxieties about her job and her relationships, and it's also helped her to focus on a novel she's been working on.

"It really helps me to put everything else aside and focus on being creative." She pauses. "Lewis Carroll used it, you know. What did you think was in that hookah the caterpillar was smoking?"

Alas, her claim about the author of *Alice's Adventures in Wonderland* is probably an urban myth. Still, I'm impressed by Julie's fervent endorsement of medical marijuana. I'm particularly impressed by the wide variety of benefits she ascribes to it, from decreased anxiety to increased creativity.

"It's made me a whole new person," she says.

As the receptionist calls her name, Julie stands up and flashes me a radiant smile. Then she strides off purposefully to pick up the renewed recommendation that she's convinced has changed her life.

Could medical marijuana really do everything that Julie says it has?

I'll give you a curated tour of what we know about what marijuana can do for us, and we'll start with the problems for which marijuana seems like an obvious treatment. Marijuana affects the brain, so we'll start with problems that are brain related, such as insomnia, anxiety, dementia, and seizures. During this tour, I'll focus on where the evidence is. I'll emphasize the medical problems for which marijuana seems to be effective. I'll leave out some problems and symptoms for which we don't yet have much evidence, but I'll give you a guide that will be more helpful than a simple laundry list of possible benefits, hypotheses, and conflicting opinions would be.

The Woman Who Played Scrabble with Herself

Of all of the medical reasons why people use marijuana, I'll start with the simplest and the most obvious: sleep. Can marijuana help us get a good night's sleep? Alice is hoping that it might.

Alice is in her midfifties, and her graying hair is pulled back in a neat bun. She's wearing a simple linen dress and no makeup or jewelry except for a plain wedding band. She could be a Mennonite housewife from eastern Pennsylvania, except that she's in a medical marijuana clinic in Southern California.

"I can't sleep," she says when I ask her why she's here. "I can't fall asleep until three or four in the morning. And even if I do, I wake up again a few hours later." Alice admits she's had this problem ever since she got married twenty-six years ago.

There's room here for a series of questions about a husband who is a restless sleeper or who snores. But I'm talking to people like Alice not as a doctor but as a visitor in a medical marijuana clinic. Besides, I'm learning that by the time people like Alice turn to medical marijuana, they've already tried most of the easy, conventional solutions. Instead, I ask her what else she has used to help her sleep.

"Oh, lots of drugs." Alice pauses, thinking. "Lots and lots. Gosh, Ambien, Ativan, Restoril, Xanax." She goes on to say she's tried over-the-counter drugs, too, such as diphenhydramine (Benadryl) and even melatonin. "Even if they got me to sleep at first, they'd wear off and I'd be wide awake in the middle of the night and staring at a Scrabble board."

Alice's doctor told her that she shouldn't just lie in bed when she couldn't sleep. She should get up and do something. So she started playing Scrabble against herself.

Other specialists recommended other remedies, including more exercise (or less), a bedtime routine, a white-noise machine, meditation, a new mattress. She shrugs. "Nothing's helped."

Then a friend mentioned that she'd started using marijuana for joint pain. "She said it worked, but she didn't like it because it made her sleepy. And so I thought, well, feeling sleepy doesn't sound so bad. Why not?"

The woman behind the counter calls Alice's name and she stands up.

"Well, here goes nothing."

She seems hopeful, but surely she's been in this position many times before, trying yet another treatment. Does she think it will help her sleep?

Alice shrugs. "Who knows? But I imagine it will be an adventure, don't you?"

I surely do. And I hope Alice finally got a good night's sleep.

The 2,700-Year-Old Drug Dealer

It's unusual for an archaeological find to be reported by international news networks, but there are exceptions. In fact, the discovery of a 2,700-year-old stash of marijuana resulted in a firestorm of publicity that was entirely predictable.[1]

In the 1990s, farmers in China's Gobi Desert stumbled across a field of unmarked graves near Turpan, in the Xinjiang-Uygur Autonomous Region. Archaeologists subsequently began to map what would turn out to be an enormous cemetery covering some 54,000 square meters. Excavations would unearth more than two thousand tombs, some more than three thousand years old.

What captured the world's interest, and what spread around the world's news outlets with an astonishing rapidity, was the report in 2008 that one of the tombs contained about a pound of marijuana. This tomb was apparently the final resting place of a male of about forty-five years old. He was interred with possessions that indicated that he enjoyed considerable social standing, and that he was a shaman.

The archaeologists discovered a large leather basket filled with something the official scientific report describes helpfully as 789 grams of "vegetative matter" which was initially assumed to be coriander. Soon they began to suspect that this vegetative matter—belonging to a shaman, the preeminent member of the prehistoric culture—might be something else. Once it was submitted for chemical analysis, it proved to be *Cannabis sativa*. That is, marijuana. Predictably, the international news went bonkers, with headlines shouting "World's oldest marijuana stash totally busted."[2]

The next step was to run a chemical analysis of the stash. There are several dozen cannabinoid molecules in marijuana, but tetrahydrocan-

nabinol (THC) and cannabidiol (CBD) are presen'
amounts, and we know much more about them than abʎ
others.

Of the two, THC is responsible for most of marijuana's effeᵪ
the brain. So, if Alice is sleeping better now thanks to marijuana, thʎ
will be because of marijuana's THC. However, it's also THC that
causes marijuana's psychoactive effects, such as feeling stoned. On the
other hand, cannabidiol won't put you to sleep, and it won't make you
high.

We know that THC is responsible for most of marijuana's effect on
the brain because of a series of experiments that Raphael Mechoulam
and colleagues did back in the 1960s. Mechoulam, an Israeli organic
chemist who is widely regarded as the grandfather of medical marijuana, was looking for a way to define the psychoactive effects of marijuana on rhesus monkeys, and he and his team studied THC.

The results of those experiments should be of considerable interest
to an insomniac like Alice. At a THC dose of 1 mg/kg, one of Mechoulam's articles reports, the monkeys became drowsy, lethargic, and had
difficulty keeping their eyes open.[3] That is, they got sleepy. At a higher
THC dose of 2 mg/kg, the monkeys became immobile and uncoordi-
nated, then they fell asleep.

A patient like Alice would be relieved to learn that these effects were
merely temporary. "The animals could, however, regain normal behavior for short periods of time if they were pinched."

What was in the 2,700-year-old marijuana stash? THC? CBD? Both?

The archaeologists didn't find much THC or CBD, but they did find
a lot of another cannabinoid: cannabinol (CBN). Cannabinol isn't normally found in large amounts in marijuana, but it's produced over time
as THC breaks down. This sample had been sitting around for a long
while. So, given how much CBN was in the sample, the archaeologists
figured that nearly three millennia ago this would have been premium,
THC-rich weed.

Second, the archaeologists also guessed that this high-octane herb
had been carefully cultivated and harvested. They noted, for instance,

that the seeds and leaves were all about the same size. (If it had been gathered from plants in the wild, there would have been much more variety.) They also found that the sample consisted entirely of buds from female plants, which are much higher in THC (i.e., marijuana that is known as sinsemilla). These plants had been selectively cultivated and harvested to maximize THC content in much the same way that growers do today.

This study offers a third interesting result, but it's one that the archaeologists don't mention. Specifically, marijuana must have been very plentiful if people were willing to drop three quarters of a kilo of perfectly good pot into a grave.

Sleepless in London

So humans have known for millennia that the ingredients of marijuana—and particularly THC—affect the brain. Of course, we don't know what that shaman used his marijuana for, and he certainly didn't know what THC is, or what it does. Maybe he was trying to get to sleep, but it seems far more likely that he was looking for that stoned feeling of euphoria that THC also produces. In fact, it wasn't until much later that we have a clear account of someone's attempt to harness THC's effect on the brain to get a good night's sleep.

In the 1840s there were many people with sleep disorders like Alice's who were trying to get a good night's sleep. One of them, Dr. John Clendinning, decided to do something about it.[4]

Clendinning, a physician at London's Marylebone Infirmary, wrote an article in which he described—and summarily dismissed—a long list of other sleep aids, including prussic acid, henbane, belladonna, and aconite.

Just in case you might be inspired to try these remedies (don't), you should know that prussic acid is the old name for hydrogen cyanide. Henbane is *Hyocyamus niger*, also known as "stinking nightshade." Belladonna is *Atropa belladonna*, or deadly nightshade. And "aconite" probably refers to plants in the genus *Aconitum*, which includes species such as wolfsbane, and which contain the toxin aconitine.

Clendinning also mentions opium, which was the most popular choice at the time, but his criticism of the humble poppy was as unsparing as his criticism of prussic acid. Opium, he tell us, tends to produce "torpor in the stomach and bowels" and it "deranges the hepatic and renal secretions." These untoward effects, he adds, are particularly prominent "in nervous females, and dyspeptic subjects of either sex."

Fortunately, he suggests an alternative: marijuana.

The centerpiece of Clendinning's argument for marijuana is the case of a forty-four-year-old "medical man." The individual's identity is not divulged, although it's worth noting that Clendinning was forty-five years old when his article was published. This coincidence, plus the inclusion of many personal details in his published report, makes it likely that the "medical man" who tried marijuana was the author himself.

Clendinning used a tincture made from the resin of marijuana buds dissolved in a small amount of alcohol. To be specific, "Squire's tincture of Indian Hemp." He—or, rather, this "medical man"—used 12 minims (that's about one grain, or 60 milligrams).

Perhaps that dose explains why Clendinning was delighted to report that this medical man finally enjoyed the effortless sleep that he'd been seeking for years. On the first trial, he observed a "slight sense of confusion and fullness in the head, with some extra activity in the action of the carotid arteries." Soon, though, he fell into "a slumber which lasted, uninterruptedly, for about six hours." More important, he noted "none of the inconveniences which opium usually produced with him."

Despite these successes with Mechoulam's rhesus monkeys and Dr. Clendinning's experimenter, there's a dire shortage of randomized controlled trials proving marijuana's value as a sleep aid, and the evidence that exists is mixed. Some studies have found benefits, while others haven't.[5]

There is some evidence that marijuana might help people like Alice get to sleep, but it appears in an unexpected place. Alice's friend tried using marijuana for joint pain and discovered that sleepiness was (for her) an unwanted side effect. It turns out that there have been several randomized controlled trials in which marijuana was used to treat pain and other symptoms in which people found that they were also able to sleep better.[6]

There has also been a lot of experience with Sativex, which is a modern version of Clendinning's tincture. It's a mix of THC and CBD dissolved in alcohol, used as a spray that's absorbed through the lining of the mouth. Although Sativex was developed initially to treat nausea, it seems to make sleeping easier for people with a variety of conditions ranging from cancer to multiple sclerosis.[7]

Because those were studies of pain and other symptoms, we can't say for sure that marijuana improves sleep. It's possible—even likely— that the THC and CBD used in those studies reduced symptoms like pain or nausea that were interfering with patients' sleep. So we don't know whether marijuana can help people with sleep disorders.

Nevertheless, based on the stories I've heard from all of the patients I've talked with, I'll go out on a limb and say marijuana looks like a pretty good way to get to sleep, especially if you're kept awake by pain or other symptoms. There are the usual cautions, of course. The dosage matters, and too much is likely to cause anxiety that will keep you awake. There's also a risk of developing tolerance over time. That's the finding of a study in which thirteen volunteers took THC by mouth on a schedule for seven days. Researchers found a small but significant reduction in sleep during that time.[8]

Still, used in moderation, marijuana is probably effective in helping people get to sleep. It's probably at least as effective as other medication. And it's certainly better than henbane.

Corned Beef, Pastrami, and the Science of Cannabinoid Receptors

How the THC in marijuana might help people like Alice get a good night's sleep is a more complicated question, but it's an important one, because the answer tells us a lot about how marijuana affects the brain. And knowing that will help us understand how it could be used to treat other symptoms like pain or nausea.

If THC makes you sleepy, then you'd think that THC molecules must bind to receptors in the brain. And there's evidence that they do.[9] Although it's difficult to map receptors directly, we can look for the traces that remain after a receptor is made.

Imagine that you walk into a deli and order a corned beef on rye. When you pay, you get a receipt. Then you hand the receipt in and you get your sandwich when it's ready. When genes make proteins, including the proteins in THC receptors, they create a messenger genetic code known as RNA. Ribonucleic acid is essentially a summary of a gene, just like a receipt for that corned beef sandwich, and like that receipt it carries instructions from the DNA in genes (the cash register in this analogy) to the place in cells where THC receptors are made (the pickup window).

Just as the deli owner can count receipts to figure out how many people are ordering corned beef compared to pastrami, it's possible to use messenger RNA to figure out what kind of receptors our cells are making. It's even possible to draw a map of where in the brain those receptors are.

Researchers found a lot of those receipts for receptors were in the brain's basal ganglia. That area works like a control center and helps to coordinate movement and balance so that movements happen in concert. It's what allows us to walk and talk and, normally, do both at the same time. It also contains a section that's responsible for "reward learning," the process by which we associate actions and consequences.

There are also lots of cannabinoid receptors in the limbic system, which is a loose collection of areas of the brain that sit beneath the outer cortex. Together, these areas are responsible for emotion and motivation, as well as memory. The hippocampus, which seems to be central in long-term memory formation, is also part of the limbic system.

There are cannabinoid receptors in the cerebellum, too. The cerebellum sits in the back of the brain, as an offshoot of the spinal column.

Indeed, it looks like a little spare brain, sticking out like a mushroom. It's responsible for coordination and balance, and especially the synthesis of the brain's control of actions and sensory input from limbs. When you reach out to turn the page of a book, for instance, it's the cerebellum that incorporates incoming information from your fingertips that tells you what you're doing.

Finally, there are cannabinoid receptors in other places in the brain, most notably in the cortex. This is the outer area of the brain—the squiggly, bumpy pattern that we're most familiar with. The cortex is responsible for higher thought as well as the control of actions.

These cannabinoid receptors appear in two types, called CB1 and CB2 receptors. The brain's neurons, which do all of our thinking and feeling, have CB1 receptors. There are also some CB2 receptors in the brain, but they only appear on microglial cells. These cells aren't responsible for thinking. Instead, they're the central nervous system's version of immune cells that clean up debris. So, if the THC in marijuana is going to help Alice get to sleep, it will probably do so by activating the CB1 receptors on neurons.

The CB1 receptors that will help her get to sleep also appear in the reproductive system in men and women. They appear in the hormonal system, too, in the thyroid, pituitary, and adrenal glands. The CB2 receptors on the glial cells in the brain also seem to play a large role in the immune system. They're particularly dense on two types of white blood cells, B lymphocytes and what are called natural killer cells, which are responsible for making antibodies and destroying foreign cells, respectively.[10] Not surprisingly, there are also many CB2 receptors wherever there are a lot of immune cells, such as in the tonsils, thymus, and spleen and in the gastrointestinal tract.

There are other cannabinoid receptors, too. Of these, perhaps the best studied are so-called vanilloid receptors, and one in particular, type 1, known as VR1. The VR1 receptor is basically a channel that lets cations (positively charged molecules like sodium) flow through the cell membrane. VR1 is particularly interesting because it's nonspecific. That is, although it can be activated by THC, it can also be turned on by heat and capsaicin, the substance that's responsible for the spiciness of chili peppers.

We'll come back to these other receptors later, as we see how marijuana might treat symptoms and problems that exist outside the brain. The important point to remember for now is that the brain has a lot of cannabinoid receptors, and most of these are CB1 receptors that bind to THC. If we're hoping that marijuana will help people with sleep disorders get to sleep, it's going to exert those effects mostly through THC.

The Dragon of Na'an

If CB1 and CB2 cannabinoid receptors are so widespread in the brain, marijuana might have other calming effects that could be useful. I'm thinking in particular about patients with dementia, who often become agitated and confused. That's a problem for their caregivers, and especially for their families. To find out whether marijuana might calm an agitated patient with dementia, I go in search of a man who has been spreading the gospel of marijuana in a very unlikely place: nursing homes.

I traveled to Tel Aviv to meet Zach Klein, a man who has administered medical marijuana to hundreds of nursing home residents with dementia and claimed success.

On my way to meet him, I discover that if you're looking for a bracing cure for the symptoms of a red-eye flight plus a seven-hour jet lag, nothing is quite as effective as a race through Tel Aviv at rush hour with a cabdriver who is blasting speed metal and singing along in Hebrew. I am now officially and irrevocably wide awake. I'm also a little unsteady on my feet as I climb out of our mobile concert hall, pay the lead singer, and stumble into an elegant restaurant.

I don't know what Zach Klein looks like, but he knows a jet-lagged traveler when he sees one. The man at the far side of the restaurant who gets up to greet me is tall, thin, and about my age. He sports a graying crew cut and long, broad sideburns that sweep down the sides of his face, making him look like an aging rockabilly singer.

Klein isn't a singer, though. Nor is he a doctor or a researcher. He's a filmmaker who became interested in medical marijuana when his mother was diagnosed with cancer back in 2000.

"Her oncologist told us, secretly, to get marijuana. It might help with the side effects of chemotherapy," he said. "Nausea . . . appetite . . . sleep . . . maybe pain."

But his mother was afraid of its effects on her brain.

"You remember riggin?"

I shake my head. Klein mimes with large, expressive hands, dropping a fist toward an upturned palm. "Your brain . . ." The fist splays into a hand in midflight. Slap. "Your brain on drugs."

Ah. Klein's English is excellent, but his accent threw me. Reagan. Ronald Reagan and his war on drugs. Apparently that war had reached across the Atlantic to scare an old lady away from medical marijuana.

There was someone Klein could turn to for advice. Raphael Mechoulam had recently won the Israel Prize, a coveted national award, for his marijuana research, and was giving public presentations of his work. Klein attended one of them and became fascinated by all of the science involved. Fascinated, and a little confused.

"It was so scientific," he says, after a pause. "Where was the talk of Bob Marley? Of joints and bongs? Instead, it was all about molecules and receptors and experiments on . . . mice."

After approaching Mechoulam at a lecture and receiving his personal assurance that marijuana was safe, Klein procured some for his mother. He saw how much better she felt after she'd used it, and he became a convert—and an evangelist.

Klein explains that many people who were starting to use medical marijuana in Israel back then had no previous experience with it. So he became certified as an instructor to teach people about doses and side effects. Part of his responsibilities included rolling joints for his patients.

Klein also did what any filmmaker would do when he was handed a story like this: he made a documentary for Israeli television (*Prescribed Grass*).

That documentary was widely viewed and well received in Israel, but its most important result came a few months after it aired. Klein got a call from a nurse who worked in a nursing home at the Na'an kibbutz (formally, Kibbutz Na'an) near Tel Aviv. She wanted advice about one of her patients who had severe dementia. The patient's family had received a marijuana license on the patient's behalf, but the nurse didn't know what to do. Legally, the patient could use marijuana, but she had dementia and couldn't actually smoke a joint.

Klein agreed to help, but when he visited the nursing home, what he found was daunting. This woman, his new pupil, was barely able to sit upright in a wheelchair, and had lost all ability to speak or understand. She would simply sit there, groaning.

"She wouldn't respond to anything," Klein says. "So I asked the nurse if I could blow some smoke on her. Like this." And he mimes taking a generous hit from a bong, and then slowly exhales imaginary marijuana smoke out toward the Mediterranean to his right.

"It was amazing. She responded immediately," he tells me. "This woman, she'd been there for a few months, and she'd never been calm and able to speak. Then she said her name, and she smiled for the first time."

He smiles, too, at the memory. "Then the nurse told me I had to stay there. She had thirty-six patients, she said. I should help them all."

They got additional licenses. Five, then ten, then more.

Although that's a lot of smoking for one person, Klein tells me he's developed a tolerance. "It's like coffee. It just becomes part of your system. I came every day to smoke, and I'd visit the first patient, then the second, then the third . . . They called me the dragon."

I'm glad that worked for him, and for the patients at Kibbutz Na'an, but I'm having trouble imagining how that method could be exported. In the United States, for instance, inspectors would have conniptions if a "marijuana instructor" showed up at a nursing home, lit up, and started blowing smoke at patients. It didn't take long, though, before someone in the kibbutz invented a Rube Goldberg–type contraption made of a glass flask, an aquarium pump, and plastic tubing. The marijuana burned and the pump pushed the resulting smoke through water and out into a balloon, from which the elderly patient inhaled. Apparently that was even more effective than Klein's secondhand smoke had been, and avoided what must have been a substantial occupational exposure for him.

He says he's seen patients with severe dementia and limbs that are bent and immobile from disuse "open like a flower." And he's seen patients with Parkinson's disease suddenly become able to write legibly. In fact, this becomes the final image in his documentary: a patient who told him to come back to film him because he'd found that, with the help of marijuana, he could sign his name again for the first time in years.

As Klein enthusiastically describes these successes while we're sitting in that café in Tel Aviv, I'm impressed, but skeptical, too. These are just stories, not the results of careful studies. Maybe these patients, and Klein himself, were somehow just fooled into thinking that they were better?

Then Klein tells me something that piques my curiosity. Not only did those patients feel better, they were able to stop some of the medications that they had been taking. Klein reviewed the charts of twenty-seven of his patients who started marijuana and found that they stopped a total of thirty-nine medications.

He knows that's not proof of cause and effect. Maybe those patients' physicians would have stopped their medications anyway, but he thinks marijuana had enough of a calming effect that some of those drugs were no longer needed.

Klein tells me the Israeli Ministry of Health has since imposed several rules, such as a requirement that any marijuana be dispensed by a pharmacist, which were too expensive for his nursing home to follow. Now the home still honors its commitment to preexisting patients, but it doesn't provide marijuana to any new patients. The nursing home's population is aging and dying, so the group of those who use it is shrinking.

As we stand up to say good-bye, Klein tells me about an eleven-year-old boy with autism who started medical marijuana recently. It hasn't cured his autism, but the boy is no longer shouting and hitting others, or himself. He's also been able to go back to school with a private teacher. I'm not surprised by Klein's parting comment to me: "I'm making a documentary."

As Good as a Motorcycle Helmet?

I'm very impressed by Klein's reports that his patients were able to stop some of their medications. Since the overuse of medications is such a problem in older people, especially in the United States, I wonder whether simply reducing medications might be of enormous value by itself. If Klein's patients were able to stop some medications and avoid some of those medications' side effects, that would be a benefit worth celebrating. A few days later I place a call to Dr. John Morley, the chief of geriatrics at Saint Louis University, and an advocate of medical marijuana for older people. Marijuana isn't legal in Missouri, so he prescribes dronabinol, a synthetic form of THC that's available by prescription.

"THC," he tells me, "does exactly what you want it to do in older people with dementia and behavioral disturbances." It's calming, for instance, and he agrees with Dr. Clendinning that it can help people sleep.

Morley also thinks it could have helped Klein's patients to stop some of their medications, particularly drugs like benzodiazepines or antipsychotics, which are often prescribed to help people sleep or to calm agitation; he's not surprised by Klein's results.

He mentions that the ingredients of marijuana might have other beneficial effects on the brain, such as reducing the inflammation that leads to damage in conditions ranging from stroke to Alzheimer's disease. Indeed, one study in rats has found that synthetic cannabinoids, including some that bind to the CB2 receptor, reduce the activity of the brain's microglial cells. (As I mentioned earlier, these are the immune cells that clean up debris between brain cells.) That study also found CB1 and CB2 receptors buried in the plaques that are associated with Alzheimer's disease.[11] So I think it's possible that marijuana might even have a role someday in the prevention or treatment of dementia.

Marijuana might also give the brain some protection after a serious accident. That's the preliminary conclusion of a study of 446 patients with a traumatic brain injury (for example, after a car accident or a fall).[12] The patients with positive blood tests for THC had a mortality rate that was only about a quarter of what it was for patients who hadn't been using marijuana. If that result is corroborated by future studies, it would mean that smoking a joint could improve your chances of survival in, say, a motorcycle accident as much as wearing a helmet does.

Of course, any speculation about cause and effect would be premature as of this writing. Maybe marijuana users had less severe accidents, or maybe they were less likely to use more dangerous drugs. And, as we'll see later in the book, there are many other reasons why marijuana and driving don't mix.

Marijuana's ingredients might even be used to treat someone who is having a stroke that's caused by a blockage of one of the brain's arteries. In 2005, researchers did experiments on mice in which one of the brain's arteries is blocked, which effectively cuts off oxygen to the brain cells that are served by that artery.[13] They found that mice that had been given CBD had a smaller area of their brains affected, and less damage.

As an interesting aside, cannabinoids might also protect against other neuronal damage. For instance, they might reduce the damage that occurs when rats are exposed to methamphetamines.[14] That is, rats given the ingredients of marijuana and methamphetamine had less brain damage than those given methamphetamine alone.

At first glance, that result seems counterintuitive. (And it certainly shouldn't be taken as advice to use two illegal drugs.) How could marijuana protect against the damage caused by strokes or methamphetamines?

One possible explanation from those studies is that the cannabinoids in marijuana reduce the activity of an enzyme called neuronal nitric oxide synthase. That enzyme produces nitric oxide, which is toxic to cells. So if cannabinoids reduce nitric oxide, injured cells may suffer less damage. Another possibility is that cannabinoids decrease inflammatory cytokines like tumor necrosis factor alpha, which is part of the body's inflammatory response. In fact, it's possible that both theories are true, and also that cannabinoids work through other mechanisms we haven't discovered yet.

These studies open up the intriguing possibility that cannabinoids such as THC and CBD might protect neurons that aren't getting enough oxygen. Oxygen deprivation occurs during a stroke, and also during a cardiac arrest or a battlefield injury when there's been massive blood loss. That is why preliminary studies like these generate enthusiasm for cannabinoids and raise hopes that they might not merely treat symptoms, but might someday be used in treating or preventing disease.

Don Quixote and Sancho Panza

I'm thinking back to something that John Morley the geriatrician told me. Marijuana isn't legal where he practices medicine, so he uses dronabinol (a synthetic form of THC) as a substitute. He also told me about THC's benefits, which he thinks are substantial.

But what about cannabidiol? So far we've seen only a few ways that CBD might be helpful. For instance, there was the study that found it might reduce the brain damage in mice after a stroke. But among all of the studies I've told you about so far, the star has been THC. In contrast, CBD seems to have only a supporting role.

In fact, their relationship is a little like that of Don Quixote and Sancho Panza in Cervantes's picaresque tale. The Don was a loopy aristocrat with odd delusions of chivalry and a skewed perception of reality that led him—among other adventures—to imagine that a windmill was a giant against which he was honor-bound to battle. Sancho, on the other hand, was the humble servant, the practical, commonsense squire.

He did his best to keep his master on the straight and narrow path, or at least to prevent him from doing too much harm to himself, or to windmills.

You can think of THC as the Don Quixote of marijuana's cannabinoids. We've seen how its receptors are scattered all over the brain, in the cortex, in the cerebellum, and in the reward centers, among other places. The fact that it binds to those widespread and diverse receptors means that it can make you goofy, confused, and even paranoid. It's responsible for the psychological effects that we associate with marijuana, such as euphoria and its "high" feeling. All those are the Quixotic effects of THC, and it's because of all of its psychological effects that THC is the cannabinoid that everyone notices.

Cannabidiol, on the other hand, is more like Sancho Panza. What's most notable about CBD is what it *doesn't* do. Specifically, it doesn't produce any of the psychoactive effects of THC. It doesn't make you feel high or paranoid, and it doesn't make you hallucinate. Like Sancho Panza, CBD does whatever it does quietly and almost invisibly.

CBD has a modulating effect. It tones down the body's—and particularly the brain's—natural responses to THC in the same way that Sancho restrained some of the Don's most exuberant nuttiness.

How CBD modulates THC's effects is interesting, because cannabidiol doesn't seem to activate the CB1 and CB2 receptors that THC binds to. That is, CBD isn't an "agonist." In the language of receptors, an agonist is a molecule that binds to a receptor and activates it. Nor is it an antagonist, which binds to a receptor and shuts it down. Instead, CBD binds weakly to CB1 or CB2 receptors and acts as an indirect antagonist. That is, it doesn't rev them up, but it doesn't shut them down, either. Just as the quiet, steady Sancho Panza reins his boss in, when CBD binds to CB1 or CB2 receptors, it prevents THC from acting at full strength.

There are some interesting hints about what this modulating effect might mean for someone who is using marijuana. It's possible that people smoking marijuana with a lot of cannabidiol might be less likely to suffer from THC's impact on thinking and memory. That finding comes from an interesting "Bring Your Own Marijuana" study of 134 experienced marijuana users.[15] Researchers gave them the chance to use their own marijuana under controlled conditions, and measured the effects of that marijuana on memory. The researchers found that marijuana's effects on memory were less severe among users whose weed was high in CBD. That is, if two people smoked joints with identical THC concentrations, the one whose joint had the higher CBD concentration fared better on memory tests. Those results are very preliminary, but they've made some researchers wonder whether CBD might ameliorate some of marijuana's possible short- or long-term effects on the brain, such as memory loss. (As we'll see, those effects aren't certain, but even a possibility of long-term memory loss is worth worrying about.)

That fits with the results of a very different laboratory study involving rhesus monkeys. Researchers used various combinations of THC and CBD, and examined the monkeys' ability to learn, remember, and perform delicate tasks. This study also found that the administration of CBD along with THC ameliorated THC's negative effects.[16]

But there's a twist. The people—and presumably the monkeys—given high-CBD marijuana still felt the euphoria and confusion that are part of being stoned. That might be because CBD enhances some of THC's effects.[17] How that happens isn't clear, but one possibility is that when CBD prevents THC from binding to its receptors, the body adapts by making more receptors. Cannabidiol may make the body's receptors more sensitive to THC. That's an interesting possibility because it might mean that CBD might let THC do its thing at lower doses.

It also seems as though CBD might work on CB2 receptors as an "inverse agonist." That's different from an antagonist or a partial agonist, which slows a receptor down. An inverse agonist causes that receptor to do the opposite of what it's supposed to do, reversing its effects. That would be like what would happen if the quiet Sancho Panza began instead to make Don Quixote *more* loopy and grandiose, inciting him to tilt at even bigger windmills.

Cannabidiol may also have other effects, through other receptors.

For instance, there's growing evidence that CBD exerts at least some of its effects on receptors for serotonin.[18] A wide variety of conditions, ranging from nausea to depression, can be treated by drugs that target serotonin receptors (e.g., ondansetron for nausea and fluoxetine, aka Prozac, for depression and obsessive-compulsive disorder).

Although we don't know nearly as much about CBD as we do about THC, it's becoming increasingly obvious that CBD has important effects on the brain and elsewhere in the body. In some ways, it's probably as important as THC, and there are some medical problems for which CBD might be more helpful than THC is.

The Girl Who Talked to Cats

Randi was a healthy baby, and the pediatrician in attendance when she was born pronounced her to be "perfect." Indeed, her parents, Cal and Cindy, had no reason to be worried. Neither of their families had any genetic diseases that they knew about, and Cindy's pregnancy had been uncomplicated.

Moreover, they were careful—almost obsessive—future parents. They were cautious, and tried to be prepared and do everything right for Cindy's first pregnancy.

I'm hearing this from Cal and Cindy while we sit in the living room of their small, neat home near San Diego. As we talk, all three of us are watching Randi, now about two and a half years old. She's a solemn child, with long hair of a golden-blond color that matches her parents' exactly. They all share the same fair skin and blue eyes, too, making them unmistakably a family.

Randi is sitting on a plush rug next to sliding glass doors that lead to the backyard. She's surrounded by stuffed animals, but her attention seems to be fixated on Buster, a very real calico cat. Randi is babbling happily in what sounds to me like nonsense sentences. The only word I catch is—improbably—"daddy."

Buster seems bemused by this unexpected promotion to fatherhood. He's watching Randi with a friendly expression, head cocked to one side. As the adults look on, Randi babbles and Buster listens intently.

"Yeah," Cal says in a voice tinged with wonder. "They have this thing. She loves telling Buster about how her day is going."

I met Cal a few days ago at a medical marijuana dispensary, and I was skeptical when he told me that he wasn't there for himself, and he wouldn't say whom he was running this errand for. But eventually he called me and said he'd be willing to talk about the reason he was in that dispensary, and that reason, it turns out, was his daughter Randi.

She was a normal baby for the first six months or so, Cindy says. Then one night, out of the blue, she had a seizure that lasted about a minute. It scared her parents, but didn't seem to leave Randi any worse off, and so Randi's pediatrician wrote it off as a onetime thing. (It's not unheard of for a child to have a single seizure, sometimes in response to a fever.) Randi had another seizure about a month later, and then another. That was not normal.

If you've ever seen a seizure, you know that a minute can seem like an hour, and that's especially true if you're watching your own child. Randi's body would become rigid, as all of her muscles seemed to tense at the same time. She looked like there were spasms coursing through every muscle in her body, and it was difficult for Cal and Cindy to tell whether she was still breathing.

Randi's doctors quickly made the diagnosis of Dravet syndrome, a rare disorder in which infants develop intractable seizures. Those seizures, and the havoc they wreak on the brain, impair neural development and learning. It's an often fatal disease that Cal tells me is as serious as cancer but much harder to treat.

Dravet syndrome is caused by a mutation in the SCN1A gene, which is responsible for the channels in a cell membrane that let sodium flow back and forth. Sodium in our bodies exists as a positively charged ion, and the concentration of sodium in a cell determines whether that cell is positively or negatively charged. Just as telephone landlines relay positive and negative charges to carry information, neurons use charges across their surface to conduct impulses. To do that, they need to be able to control positive ions such as sodium. But if they lose control of those ions, the result is a little like what happens when lightning strikes a telephone pole, disrupting signals and frying circuits.

When Randi turned two, Cal says, everything changed. "It was as if someone turned a dial in her head, cranking up whatever was going on in there." Soon Randi was having a seizure almost every day, and those seizures went on for ten or fifteen minutes.

They went to specialists, who tried seemingly endless combinations of seizure medications. Some seemed to help, Cindy says, but it was hard to be sure if they really were helping. And any improvements were just a temporary reprieve.

Then, about three months ago, Cal and Cindy started giving Randi the marijuana-based oil that he got from the dispensary where I met him. This oil is made from those parts of the plant that have high concentrations of THC and CBD. A joint usually has less than 5 percent THC and CBD, but a drop of the oil they're using might have as much as 50 percent CBD.

For Cal and Cindy, their decision to try the oil really wasn't much of a choice. "We'd tried a dozen other medicines," Cal told me. "Easily a dozen. And all of them had side effects and warnings."

Such as?

"Oh, a low white blood cell count, anemia, confusion, delirium, muscle pain, bleeding gums, lack of coordination."

They decided that they wanted oil that had high concentrations of CBD, and as little THC as possible. Although they told me that neither of them used marijuana recreationally, they knew about its psychological effects, and they didn't want to inflict those effects on their toddler. But they'd also done enough research on the Internet and in chat rooms of Dravet parents to know that they could avoid those psychological effects by using CBD oil. That is what they found.

"It's pure CBD," Cindy tells me. "No THC at all."

Remember, it's THC that's responsible for the "high" of marijuana, so Cal and Cindy wanted oil that wouldn't inflict any of those effects on their daughter. To make sure, they had it tested by a laboratory. Those tests showed that the oil was 57 percent CBD and less than 1 percent THC. Finally, Cal and Cindy discussed Randi's options with her pediatrician and a neurologist who specializes in childhood epilepsy.

"They didn't actually tell us we should use it," Cal says. "They didn't really recommend it. It was more like they gave us permission. They said it might be OK, if we really wanted to try."

So they did, at a very low dose at first. Just a few drops mixed with applesauce. They guessed they were giving about 25 milligrams of CBD, twice a day. That's a modest dose, even for a small child.

"At first, we weren't looking for it to help at all," Cindy says. "We just hoped it wouldn't hurt her." She adds that they were ready to stop at the first sign of trouble. But they didn't encounter any.

Gradually they increased the dose to about 100 milligrams, given twice a day. That's when Randi's seizures started to wane.

"This stuff is miracle oil," Cindy says.

"It wasn't magic," Cal cautions. "It wasn't like someone flipped a switch. But she just . . . missed a couple of days. We hardly noticed at first."

And in between? Did they notice any changes in Randi's personality? Or her behavior?

I'm wondering whether she was more sleepy, or maybe confused. Even at very low concentrations of THC, Randi was still getting some. But Cal and Cindy say that Randi started showing an interest in the world around her in a way that she hadn't since her seizures started. She also began telling Buster the cat about her day.

The Science of "Miracle Oil"

As I learn more about Dravet syndrome, I realize that Randi's story isn't unusual. Parents are often desperate to find something—anything—that might help their child. Her experience with multiple medications is very typical of what other kids endure. In one survey, the parents of nineteen children with intractable seizures said they'd tried an average of a dozen medications before considering the oil that Cal and Cindy tried.[19] Researchers have explored the use of cannabinoids for intractable seizures for more than forty years. Indeed, it was Raphael Mechoulam who did some of the earliest studies, back in the 1970s.[20]

Could THC and CBD prevent seizures? They might. Early animal studies have found that cannabinoids do seem to be effective in preventing or reducing seizures.[21] Interestingly, studies of mice have also found that these antiseizure effects don't rely on the CB1 and CB2 receptors that we've talked about so far.[22] Cannabidiol in particular may work by means of other receptors that we don't understand very well yet.[23]

Whether CBD by itself reduces seizures in people remains an open question. In 2012, a group of researchers searched the literature, looking for any evidence they could find for the use of CBD in seizures.[24] They found a grand total of forty-eight patients in whom the use of CBD for seizures had been carefully described in medical journals. Unfortunately, the methods used in those studies varied so widely that the researchers couldn't be sure whether CBD had any effect at all. The best they could say was that CBD in doses of 200 to 300 milligrams daily seemed to be safe.

Although we don't know whether CBD is effective, it's probably no more harmful than the dozens of other drugs that kids like Randi are taking. And Cal and Cindy are convinced that the CBD oil they've procured is helping her. Many other parents of kids with Dravet syndrome are equally enthusiastic. They must know what they're talking about, right?

To find out, I contacted a neurologist named Orrin Devinsky. He's the director of New York University Langone Medical Center's Comprehensive Epilepsy Center, and I'd heard that he thinks that CBD might be effective in treating Dravet syndrome. He tells me that when he announced that he was opening a randomized, controlled trial that would give these kids access to cannabinoids, the response was overwhelming.

In that trial, Devinsky is using CBD, just as Cal and Cindy are. He isn't certain how it might work, although his best guess is that it might bind to a receptor called GPR-55 and change the calcium concentrations inside brain cells.[25]

"GPR" is shorthand for G-protein coupled receptors. That is, GPR-55 is like CB1 and CB2: it has a similar structure but it behaves differently, and has different effects inside the cell. GPR-55 is just one of a growing list of endocannabinoid receptors such as GPR-18 and GPR-119, and probably others we haven't discovered yet.

Devinsky is testing CBD instead of THC because he thinks that as many as 80 percent of kids might respond to CBD, compared with perhaps 60 percent of kids who get THC. And, as Cal and Cindy told me, CBD is probably also safer in young children than THC, which has psychoactive effects. Devinsky also thinks that in some cases THC might make seizures worse. So, even if CBD isn't 100 percent effective for all kids, it seems to offer the best chance of benefit and at least it won't make them worse.

Although Devinsky doesn't want to stake out an opinion before he has the data, he's been impressed by the stories from parents like Cal and Cindy. It's those stories—lots of them—that induced him to conduct this trial for kids with Dravet syndrome.

However, there's a warning you need to keep in mind in thinking about the potential benefits of marijuana for seizures—and indeed for most medical conditions. Whether marijuana (or any treatment) "works" will depend on what the alternatives are. Even if a given drug isn't very effective, it may be the best treatment that mainstream medicine can offer for that particular problem at the time, so we'll say that (for now) it works. However, as other better, safer treatments are developed, that drug will start to look less attractive. Eventually, doctors will set it aside.

Consider this cautionary tale: In the 1970s, marijuana was commonly used to treat glaucoma, a condition in which pressure builds up inside the eye, causing pain and a loss of vision. Although marijuana *is* effective in treating glaucoma, new drugs have proven to be much better, so marijuana is no longer recommended.[26] Thus, as new drugs are developed, our verdict on whether marijuana is effective in treating seizures or other problems may look very different five or ten years from now.

The Man Who Couldn't Forget

So far, marijuana's benefits are looking impressive. The use of THC or CBD to treat seizures is still just a theory, but marijuana does seem to be able to help people get to sleep, and might calm the agitation caused by dementia. I wonder whether marijuana might be used to help a patient who has a mix of many psychological symptoms—someone like Tomas.

Tomas tells me he doesn't go out much these days. After he was kidnapped several years ago while working in Mexico, he was plagued by frequent panic attacks, sometimes half a dozen times a day. When those attacks hit, he was paralyzed and unable to function. He would sweat enough to soak his shirt, his heart raced, and he felt as though he was suffocating. If he was at home with his wife he'd lock himself in the bathroom, and if he was out with friends he retreated to the backseat of their car. Soon he didn't want to go out anymore, and he and his wife lost touch with their friends.

Tomas also had recurrent nightmares about the kidnapping, and the beatings he received as it became apparent that his family wouldn't be able to pay his ransom. Even during the day, he was anxious all the time. Eventually his wife convinced him to see a psychiatrist, who diagnosed post-traumatic stress disorder (PTSD).

That diagnosis led to what would soon become a long list of medications. Tomas recalls being prescribed Xanax, Lexapro, chorazepam, Wellbutrin, Seronex, Prozac, Lunesta, clonazepam, and Ambien, among others. He recalls that the side effects of those medications were terrible, especially the sexual side effects. "You know that's the last thing we needed, my wife and me," he says. "All of these panic attacks and anxiety, and the problems in the bedroom . . . It was bad."

He's particularly dismissive of all of the doctors he visited. "I lost all my faith in medicine. I mean, no offense?"

None taken.

"Those doctors, they either didn't believe me, or they thought that I should be better by now. They just wanted to give me a prescription. It's like writing a prescription is their answer to everything."

Tomas mentions that he tried desensitization therapy, too, in which he was asked to mentally relive the experiences that left him emotionally scarred, in a safe and controlled environment. That worked for a little while, but soon his symptoms returned. Eventually, he tried marijuana at the suggestion of one of his friends, who gave him a joint. "It was amazing. A whole different world. It calmed me down for a whole evening and I snagged the first good night's sleep I've had in years. The anxiety got better, too."

Soon he started using marijuana regularly. "Now I can go out, and we can have people over to our apartment. It used to be that every stranger was a threat. I wouldn't let anyone get close to me."

I realize that he and I are sitting in a small, windowless room, and the door behind him is closed. I point at the door. A couple of months ago?

Tomas nods. "Yeah, a couple of months ago I wouldn't be here with you. Or if I was, I'd be freaking out and sweating and looking for a way out."

The real turning point, though, was when his wife noticed that he was more like his old self.

"We were out at a bar with some friends, and she pulled me aside and told me I seemed different. I looked like I used to, she said. That's when I knew I'd found something."

Treatment or Band-Aid?

A diagnosis of post-traumatic stress disorder is made when someone suffers a traumatic event and then reexperiences that event, becomes anxious, and avoids situations that could trigger a reexperience. Tomas is more or less a textbook case. And outside of his case, there's some preliminary evidence that marijuana might relieve PTSD symptoms. In one study, researchers talked with people like Tomas who were using marijuana to treat their PTSD.[27] First, the researchers asked a series of diagnostic questions to confirm that the person truly did have PTSD. They were looking for symptoms that define post-traumatic stress, such as distressing memories of an event, flashbacks, nightmares, as well as feelings of numbness, anxiety, or anger. Then they asked those ques-

tions based on how the person used to feel, before he or she started using marijuana. The people they surveyed scored much worse on those
questions when they recalled how they used to be.

Memory isn't perfect, and it's possible that they remembered their
condition as being worse than it really was. But there's another, more
convincing study that makes me optimistic that marijuana might be
useful in cases of PTSD. That study enrolled twenty-nine Israeli combat veterans who were given joints containing a whopping 23 percent
THC.[28] (Concentrations in a typical joint are more like 5 percent.)
Their post-traumatic stress symptoms, measured with questions similar to those used in the study I just mentioned, decreased by almost
half.

Even more promising are some laboratory studies of marijuana's ingredients and their effects on PTSD. Not PTSD symptoms, but the disorder itself. These studies have tested marijuana in desensitization
therapy, based on the idea that if you keep exposing someone to something they're afraid of, but without the negative consequences, the bad
memories will fade. Desensitization therapy worked for Tomas at first,
but his symptoms came back.

Fear memories seem to be difficult to get rid of entirely. So they sit
there, waiting for the wrong "trigger" to cue them up. But marijuana
might help. In a small trial that enrolled people without a history of
PTSD, volunteers were "conditioned" by showing them colored squares,
some of which (the yellow and blue ones) were followed by a burst of
very loud white noise through headphones.[29] Not surprisingly, subjects
developed an anxiety response to the colored squares, as measured by
change in skin conductance.

(This is the same test that's used in lie detectors. Because perspiration increases the skin's ability to conduct a very low-voltage current, a
drop in skin conductance is an indicator of perspiration. And that's an
indicator of anxiety.)

The red squares weren't followed by loud noise, and so they didn't
make subjects anxious. The following day, some subjects were given
THC (7.5 milligrams by mouth), while others got a placebo. Then they

were all shown the blue squares without the noise, to extinguish their anxiety responses. In the study's final test, those who were given THC had smaller increases in anxiety in response to the blue squares compared to subjects who got a placebo. Their response to that anxiety-provoking cue was still there, but had been reduced.

Interestingly, another measure of emotional memory—subjects' expectations of that loud noise—wasn't affected. People expected that loud noise, but it didn't bother them. It seems as though the subjects who were given the THC were better able to forget to be afraid of those blue squares.

Christine Rabinak, the study's lead author, explained to me that THC's CB1 receptors are very dense in two areas of the brain: the prefrontal cortex and the amygdala. These areas are involved in learning, particularly "emotional learning." That term refers to mental associations that are formed under periods of intense emotion, as in the setting of trauma. THC seems to act on the areas of the brain where emotional memories are formed, stored, and resurrected. Rabinak thinks that THC might be useful in treating PTSD—not just in relieving PTSD symptoms, but in actually treating the underlying disorder. For instance, it might be a complement to the desensitization treatment that Tomas used, making it more effective.

It's admittedly a long way from studies of colored squares to the sorts of symptoms Tomas was experiencing, and Rabinak is quick to acknowledge that there's a lot that we don't know, such as what the optimal dose of THC might be. She gave her subjects 7.5 milligrams as an educated guess. "You want to give enough to have an effect," she says. "But you don't want to give so much that you reduce anxiety." That, she explains, could cloud the results of the exposure therapy, because people who are completely and utterly mellow don't get anxious during treatment. At even higher doses, she reminds me, THC can cause anxiety.

Rabinak has other questions, too. How often should THC be given? When should it be given? What will it do outside of her trials? Will people who don't respond to exposure therapy begin to respond with some help from THC? Rabinak wants answers to those questions before she even thinks about recommending THC for patients like Tomas.

There's another, bigger reason why she's concerned that lots of people like Tomas are using marijuana to treat their PTSD.

"People come up to me when I give talks and they tell me how much marijuana helps them. Lots of people with anxiety or PTSD self-medicate. They feel anxious and they use it. Sure, that makes them feel better, but it doesn't fix the underlying problem."

Rabinak is hopeful that her research will find a way to use THC very differently. She wonders whether it might be a way to make exposure therapy more effective, and more long lasting, in much the same way that we use a combination of radiation therapy and chemotherapy for cancer. Together, maybe THC and exposure therapy are more effective than exposure therapy alone.

Another Victory for Sancho Panza

Even in theory, there's a problem with using THC—or marijuana—to treat fear and anxiety, and it's a problem that Christine Rabinak alluded to when she explained why she chose the low 7.5-milligram dose.

THC in low doses can be calming, as John Morley and Zach Klein have learned, but in higher doses, one of the most common side effects of THC is anxiety. The wrong dose might actually make symptoms worse. The fear responses of PTSD are bad enough, as Tomas knows; add more anxiety and paranoia, and you have a very unpleasant mix.

We shouldn't give up on marijuana as a treatment for PTSD simply because it could increase anxiety. After all, there are plenty of other (legal) drugs that exacerbate the symptoms they're intended to treat. Benzodiazepines such as Valium are used for their calming effects, but sometimes they cause an increase in agitation. Opioids like morphine in very high doses can also make people extremely sensitive to pain.

Besides, there might be a solution. In a study that was similar to Rabinak's, researchers used colored images and shocks to condition a fear response in forty-eight subjects.[30] Instead of giving subjects THC, as Rabinak did, these researchers used CBD—the quiet Sancho Panza to THC's Don Quixote. For people who were given CBD, their fear response declined faster than it did for those people who received a placebo.

CBD won't make you feel high, nor does it cause the sort of anxiety that THC does, so it might reduce anxiety without the risk of a paradoxical reaction. Patients like Tomas wouldn't have to worry that the drug they're taking to reduce their anxiety might actually produce a panic attack.

In another study, college students were put through a session in which they had to give a speech, and then they watched themselves on a video monitor. That's a task that would produce anxiety in anyone, especially for those volunteers in the sample who had social anxiety disorder.[31] The main result of that study was that the students with social anxiety disorder were much less anxious if they were given 600 milligrams of CBD.

But how does it work? Remember that CBD doesn't really have much of an effect on the CB1 and CB2 receptors in the brain, which appear on neurons and microglial cells. One theory is that it binds to other receptors in the brain, like serotonin receptors or the GPR-55 receptors that Orrin Devinsky is interested in. But we really don't know yet.

In another small study, ten people with social anxiety disorder were given either 400 milligrams of CBD or a placebo. Then they switched, so everyone got CBD.[32] As the researchers expected, CBD reduced subjects' anxiety. The researchers took a look at subjects' brains in a functional MRI scanner, which gives a real-time view of the parts of the brain that are most active. Those scans found that CBD caused reductions in brain activity in the areas of the brain most associated with pathological levels of anxiety.

Therefore, CBD doesn't have a general calming effect. Instead, it seems to be acting in a very focused way on the circuits of the brain that are responsible for heightened anxiety.

Based on all of these studies, it seems likely that Tomas probably was getting some relief from his symptoms, and it's possible that at least some of those effects are attributable to CBD. That's good news, but Rabinak's warning is concerning, too. Tomas wasn't really treating his underlying PTSD; he was treating some of its most prominent symptoms. If Rabinak is right, he'll need to keep using marijuana for a long time. Still, Tomas would probably say that it's done more than any prescription drug has done for him, and that the relief it offers is plenty to be thankful for.

The Truth Behind the Buzz

One of the biggest—and most exciting—surprises for me in this chapter has been the realization that marijuana doesn't just make you high. Its ingredients, THC and CBD, have very specific effects on our brains. Even better is the fact that CBD might offer some of those benefits without the "high" feeling that some people would rather avoid.

Based on the studies I've shown you, I think it's reasonable to assume that, in the right dose, marijuana will probably help Alice get to sleep, and it certainly seems to calm the agitation and confusion of people with dementia. As for the treatment of seizures, the jury's still out. At best, we have lots of reports by parents like Cal and Cindy who have seen favorable results. Still, CBD seems like the best option most of these kids have. Especially now that oils are available that are almost pure CBD and virtually no THC, there's no real risk that kids will get stoned. As a scientist, I want to see Orrin Devinsky's trial results before rendering a verdict. However, if I were a parent of a child with Dravet syndrome, I'd probably make the same decision that Cal and Cindy did, secure in the knowledge that CBD alone seems safe, and that it's probably safer than a lot of other medications that they'd tried.

I'm also hopeful about Tomas and his PTSD. I'd like to believe that he finally found a treatment that works for him, and it certainly seems to work. Marijuana seems to be more effective than other medications, and less toxic. So I hope it continues to work for him and that he does well. Personally, I'd like to see evidence from a randomized controlled trial that marijuana is safe and effective for people like him, not just for a couple of weeks but for years.

Overall, though, it seems that medical marijuana is looking much more promising than I thought it would. I've seen some pretty convincing evidence that it's effective, and the experiments with pure THC and CBD offer an enticing hint of what might be possible someday.

3

The Woman with Knives in Her Neck: Marijuana's Benefits for the Body

I've shown you some benefits of medical marijuana that seem to be real, or at least plausible. People using it for insomnia or anxiety or even seizures might be on the right track. At least there is some evidence to support those uses. And these uses are plausible because those symptoms exist in the brain, and if there's one thing we know for sure about marijuana, it's that this stuff affects the brain.

However, I'm looking at a colorful brochure that makes much grander claims about marijuana's usefulness. This document—really a small book—is designed as a sort of infomercial for a medical marijuana clinic in San Diego. Its claims are broad, diverse, and strain credulity.

There is the claim, for instance, of "relief of headaches and migraines."

Also, "aches and pains." The brochure mentions nausea, too, as well as diarrhea, constipation, and urinary incontinence.

"Menstrual and pre-menstrual pain" are listed, as well as "painful sexual intercourse" and the all-encompassing "female troubles."

There's much more. Apparently marijuana helps "those struggling with cancer treatment," as well as those with neuropathy and "inflammatory conditions."

The list of promised benefits is much longer than that. Indeed, it seems to encompass virtually every malady known to medicine. (Also, some, like "neural imbalance," whose existence I don't remember learning about in medical school.)

Which of these medical benefits are real and which are just advertising?

That's an important question, because I've met many patients who are using marijuana for a wide range of symptoms, such as pain and nausea and weight loss.

Some of these symptoms are related to what goes on in the brain, of course. But they're also at least partly outside the brain. One use—treating cancer—doesn't have much to do with the brain at all.

Could marijuana be used to treat these, too? That's more speculative, because we know much less about marijuana's effects on the rest of the body than we do about its effects on the brain. And we know less about cannabinoid receptors elsewhere in the body. But many people are using marijuana for symptoms like nausea and pain and appetite loss, so it's worth investigating.

The Woman with Knives in Her Neck

There is no "typical" medical marijuana patient. The marijuana clinics that I've visited have encompassed a wide swathe of society, and people like Alice and Tomas are living proof of the diversity of this population. However, my first thought when I meet Rachel in this particular waiting room is that she doesn't belong here.

Rachel is in her early forties, blond, and wearing a crisply tailored deep-blue suit that looks like it's made of expensive silk. Just for comparison, the guy sitting next to her in the waiting room is a skinny, unshaven lad wearing baggy shorts, a tank top, and flip-flops. Rachel looks like she's taking a well-earned break from a board meeting. Later I find out she's the co-owner of a large chain of boutiques.

She tells me that she's used marijuana recreationally since her early teens. But it wasn't until a year ago that she started turning to marijuana for other reasons. A year ago she was at the site for a new store when a piece of construction equipment fell on her. The impact fractured her cervical spine, initially leaving her paralyzed. After a month in the hospital—much of that time spent in the neurosurgical ICU— her spine was stabilized and she was able to walk and talk again.

When pieces of her spine had broken, they'd damaged some of the nerves that emerge from the spinal cord. Those damaged nerves caused unpredictable episodes of sharp pain. Rachel tells me the pain feels like knives are stabbing her neck and shooting down her arms as far as her fingers.

"They hit me when I move the wrong way, but I can't avoid them. They just . . . happen."

Those attacks were so severe, and so unpredictable, they scared her away from regular exercise. Eventually she avoided walking her dog or even doing the dishes because she was afraid that the wrong move would bring on another lightning strike. The drugs her doctors prescribed didn't help much, and opioids like morphine made her feel "drugged." She tried several different opioids, but couldn't stand them, so she turned to marijuana.

Rachel tells me that once she started using it, two things happened. First, as she'd hoped, the bouts of pain became less severe, and, as that happened, she became less afraid of the next episode. She began to exercise more, she took her corgi for long walks, and then she started seeing her trainer again for light aerobic workouts. As she did that, it seemed that the spells of pain got less frequent.

She uses a marijuana-based oil like what Cal and Cindy gave to Randi, but Rachel's oil has a lot of THC, and she uses it in a vape pen. These devices are like e-cigarettes, except that they deliver THC and CBD instead of nicotine. Rachel says she uses her vape pen "all day."

How many times?

Rachel thinks carefully. "A dozen."

I'm not sure what my expression reveals, but whatever it is causes her to reevaluate, although not in the direction I expected.

"Maybe two dozen?"

I'm having trouble imagining how twenty-four doses of mind-scrambling THC might affect a daily routine that involves managing a chain of clothing stores. But Rachel seems bemused by my questions.

"Well, we opened two new stores in the last three months. I must be doing something right."

Brain Bubble Wrap

To find out if the ingredients of marijuana could be used to treat pain, I track down a researcher who has thought a lot about this question.

Barth Wilsey is tall and baby-faced, with short-cropped hair and the peaceful gravity of a Buddhist monk. He's an anesthesiologist by training, and he's done some of the most interesting research I've seen on marijuana and pain. As I tell him Rachel's story, he listens patiently, nodding. He tells me it was people like Rachel who led him to a career of research on the uses of marijuana for pain. Wilsey recalls how, two decades ago, when he was working a pain fellowship in San Francisco, many of his patients got marijuana through a buyer's club in Oakland. They told him it was the only thing they'd found that worked for them. "That," he says, "really grabbed my attention."

Then he says something that grabs *my* attention.

"Those people all had neuropathic pain, like Rachel did."

What he means is that they had a very specific type of pain. Neuropathic pain isn't caused by an injury, like arthritis or a broken bone, that's stimulating normal nerves. Neuropathic pain is caused by the nerves themselves. To understand neuropathic pain, it helps if you think about the way that electronic devices like pagers and cell phones work. When I was a resident, two of us had to carry the "code pager" at all times. This was the pager that would go off if someone had a cardiac arrest anywhere in the hospital. Because these devices were so impor-tant, they were designed to withstand the apocalypse. To make them especially dependable, these pagers operated on local emergency radio channels that were reliable but were filled with static. And that static manifested as the triple beep of a code. Every once in a while, a pager would spring to life, emitting an unintelligible squawk and three beeps that would send a confused resident scrambling for the door, until it became apparent that it was just a false alarm.

That's how neuropathic pain happens. An injury to a nerve creates static, but nerves don't know how to interpret static any more than those pagers knew how to interpret it. Instead, nerves that carry pain signals interpret static just like they interpret any signal: as pain. Just as those emergency pagers interpreted static as an emergency and let loose a bloodcurdling beep, nerves that carry pain assume that static rep-resents a painful stimulus, and that's what they tell the brain.

Wilsey is particularly interested in Rachel's case because he thinks that if marijuana can treat pain, it's most likely to be effective in treat-ing neuropathic pain.

Wilsey believes it is effective. He mentions several studies that he and others have done.[1] He's also been impressed by what his patients told him when he asked them to abstain from marijuana for a month before they enrolled in his clinical trials. He wanted to give them a chance to get any preexisting cannabinoids out of their system, because THC or CBD can be stored in the body for days and even weeks. "We had a ter-rible time recruiting patients," he recalls. "They just couldn't wait a month, they were having so much pain. They had to start using medical marijuana again." He dropped that waiting period down to a week.

How does marijuana relieve pain? This is where things get interest-ing, because what Wilsey tells me is not what I've been expecting.

"You've got your glial cells," he says. "They're the predominant cell type in the brain."

As I explained in the previous chapter, THC binds to CB2 recep-tors on glial cells, which are immune cells in the brain. So how could they be involved in treating pain? I admit somewhat sheepishly that I didn't think that glial cells *did* anything. Sure, they have some sort of immune function. But mostly I've always thought of them as sort of . . .

"Bubble wrap," Wilsey says.

Bubble wrap?

"People used to think of glial cells as the bubble wrap of the brain. They're cells that the important neurons are packed in. Helpful, even essential. But inert."

I love this analogy, but I learn that it's not true.

Wilsey explains that glial cells aren't just structural, and they're not just immune cells. They may have a big role in pain management.

He's not sure yet what that role might be. One theory is that glial cells have some sort of modulating effect on neurons, or perhaps they work through cytokines, which are molecules that coordinate the body's response to inflammation. Whatever the mechanism, Wilsey is convinced that these cells are much more than bubble wrap.

Not only is Wilsey more interested in glial cells than neurons, he's also more interested in CBD than he is in THC. Just as CBD might be effective in treating anxiety and seizures, he thinks it might be effective in treating pain, particularly neuropathic pain. As evidence, he points out that the prescription drug dronabinol (pure THC) that John Morley used for agitation in dementia doesn't seem to work very well for pain, but marijuana that contains THC and CBD does seem to work.

If that's true—or if it might be true—then we should rethink how we do clinical trials of marijuana for pain. Most trials, Wilsey says, focus on marijuana's THC content. CBD content, in contrast, is mostly an afterthought, but Wilsey wants to do trials of marijuana that contain more CBD and less THC, a ratio of 5:1 or higher. He thinks that marijuana with a lot of CBD might lead to greater pain relief, and perhaps fewer psychological side effects.

If CBD is more valuable than we thought, it's also possible that THC isn't as necessary as we'd assumed. Wilsey tells me that his studies have pushed THC levels lower and lower. Initially he used marijuana that had a THC concentration of 7 percent, then he reduced that to 3.5 percent, and then to as low as 1.3 percent. In each subsequent study, he found as much pain relief, but fewer psychological side effects.

What's next? If marijuana is useful in treating neuropathic pain, it could be useful in other conditions that damage nerves. There's some evidence that THC and CBD reduce muscle stiffness in patients with multiple sclerosis (MS), a progressive neurologic condition that causes progressive weakness, neuropathic pain, muscle stiffness, and spasms.[2] Another study found that patients who received a mix of THC and CDB had fewer muscle spasms.[3] That mix also seems to be effective in reducing so-called central pain, which is pain that is caused when circuits in the brain misfire.[4]

The ingredients of marijuana might also slow the progression of MS. That's the optimistic conclusion of a laboratory study of mice that used a virus to mimic an MS-like syndrome.[5] The study found that CBD reduced inflammation by slowing white blood cells' response, and by disrupting their ability to stick to the walls of blood vessels. Even better, CBD reduced MS's long-term effects on movement and coordination.

There's still a lot we don't know, and not all evidence points to a benefit. A randomized, controlled trial of dronabinol (THC) didn't find that it slowed worsening of the disease.[6] Further, although THC and CBD might relieve pain and muscle spasms,[7] their use might be associated with problems of thinking and memory.[8] So, marijuana's benefits are still uncertain, and there may be risks of using it, too.

Neuropathic pain is Wilsey's specialty, but I wonder what he thinks about "nociceptive" pain. That's the kind of pain you feel if you pull a muscle or break a leg. It's also the kind of pain that I often see in my patients with advanced cancer.

Wilsey shrugs. "We're not really sure, but there's reason to think there might not be much benefit."

He tells me about studies that have used a common laboratory test of pain. You expose volunteers' skin to a piece of metal that's been heated to a temperature that most of us would agree is uncomfortable (about 45 degrees Celsius, or about 113 degrees Fahrenheit). That's their "pain threshold." Then you see whether a drug lets people tolerate a higher temperature without squirming. Wilsey says that marijuana doesn't seem to increase pain thresholds as much as some other drugs, such as morphine.[9]

What that means for patients like Rachel isn't clear, nor do we know how cannabinoids might be used someday to treat pain, but there is reason to suspect that they might play a much larger role in pain than we realize. Wilsey says that we don't know much about the effect of cannabinoids in "regular" nociceptive pain because there just haven't been many studies. Most of the research has been on neuropathic pain because that kind of pain can be very difficult to treat. Rachel had been to multiple specialists and had received countless drugs. Those drugs either didn't work or caused unacceptable side effects, or both, so she was ready to try anything.

On the other hand, patients with more common nociceptive pain have numerous treatment options. There's acetaminophen (Tylenol), which has been around for decades because it works, as well as nonsteroidals like ibuprofen (Motrin) and opioids like morphine. They all work well, so there's not a lot of pressure to come up with another new drug to treat nociceptive pain.

As Wilsey says good-bye, I'm thinking that maybe Rachel was onto something. There's research evidence that what she was doing works, and there's even growing evidence about *how* it works. That's as much as we can say about most drugs, and more than we can say about many.

Less Pain *and* Less Morphine?

There's one more element of Rachel's story that I'm curious about. She wasn't using marijuana just because it helped her; as with other patients I've met, she also wanted to avoid the side effects of opioids like morphine.

Many of my patients would prefer to replace their opioids with something else if they could. Opioids can cause nausea and dizziness, especially at first. They cause constipation, too, often requiring the use of laxatives every day. And they can make you sleepy, forgetful, and sometimes confused.

Could marijuana help someone to reduce his dose of opioids, or stop them altogether?

To try to answer that question, I seek out Jonathan Gavrin, a physician who has given more opioids to patients in a day than most doctors give in a year. Like Wilsey, he's an anesthesiologist. But he's also a palliative care physician who knows a lot about pain management. Gavrin is wiry and compact, with short hair and narrow, rectangular glasses. He looks a little like a younger, fitter Kevin Spacey.

I tell him about Rachel and her desire to avoid opioids.

"Oh, sure. I know that's true." Gavrin proceeds to tell me about his bad experiences with opioids and other drugs after he underwent a knee replacement a couple of years ago.

"They made me sick. Really sick. Hated it." He pauses. "No euphoria, though. They didn't make me feel good. Just crappy." He laughs. "I got ripped off."

So if marijuana could reduce the need for opioids?

"That would be great. We don't want our patients drowning in a pharmacological soup."

Yet we do inflict this on patients like Rachel, Tomas, and Alice. We add drugs on top of drugs, and Rachel was by no means the only victim of a doctor's prescription pad.

Gavrin laughs again. "Well, of course. We desperately want to make people feel better. So we do everything we can to help. That's why we've developed such a drug culture. It's hard to see people suffer, so we reach for a prescription pad. Maybe we get lucky with the first drug, but sometimes not, and we add, and add."

I tell Gavrin about a study that was done in San Francisco by Donald Abrams.[10] He wanted to find out whether marijuana might complement—and perhaps reduce—opioids like morphine. He wasn't trying to get people off opioids per se, but he knew that his patients often wanted to reduce their opioids if they could.

That study enrolled twenty-one patients, all of whom had pain for which they were taking scheduled opioids such as morphine or oxyco-done. Although some had neuropathic pain, many had nociceptive pain. Abrams found that patients who were given marijuana had less pain, and they had the same blood levels of opioids. Marijuana might work together with opioids to give better pain relief, and that creates the possibility that marijuana might help patients get what Rachel wanted: comfort without the side effects of opioids.

"That," Gavrin says, "would be cool."

The Man Who Looked Fabulous on Chemo

If marijuana might be effective in treating pain—or at least neuropathic pain—are there other symptoms that it could be used for? I'm thinking about all of the distressing symptoms that cause suffering in my pa-tients, and pretty close to the top of that list is nausea.

It's hard to see how marijuana could be useful in treating nausea. It's not a psychological symptom like insomnia or anxiety, and it doesn't involve damaged nerves the way that neuropathic pain does. But I've met at least one patient who's convinced that marijuana is the best treatment he's found.

Jason is in his late twenties, and painfully thin, with a crew cut and carefully trimmed beard. Despite his diminutive frame, he walks with a big-guy swagger that's complemented by elaborate tattoos that twine up both arms and around his neck.

Jason tells me he was diagnosed with non-Hodgkin's lymphoma about a year ago. Since then he's suffered through a lengthy period of intensive chemotherapy that's left him struggling with fatigue, weak-ness, and hair loss, and it caused the worst nausea he'd ever experienced.

"It was relentless, you know? No matter what my doctor gave me, I was sure that I was going to spend the next week leaning over a bucket."

Unlike most other patients I've spoken with, Jason didn't try mari-juana on his own.

"My dad was in corrections. So I grew up thinking that marijuana was bad. It would get you stoned, then addicted."

What changed his mind, eventually, was the recommendation of his oncologist, who couldn't find any other drugs that would work.

So did it help?

"Oh yeah. I was like a different person."

I'm hearing that phrase a lot. People say they feel like a different person, or others tell them, as Tomas's wife did, that they seem more like themselves.

It took a little bit of practice, but pretty soon Jason knew how much to take and how to take it. A couple of hits on a vape pen during chemo worked wonders. Then he smoked a joint at home.

"I went from puking for a week to sometimes not at all." He shakes his head as if he can't quite believe it.

"Do you know what clinched the deal for me? It was the chemo nurses. I came in the second day of chemo and they were expecting me to be all miserable and withdrawn, but I was doing OK. They said I looked *fabulous*. I mean, that's not a word anyone would ever use to describe me, but that's what they said."

He pauses. "Look, you take care of people with cancer, right?"

I nod.

"Well, how often can you honestly say one of your patients on chemo looks fabulous?"

Not often.

But what about his classes? His schoolwork? We know that THC impairs concentration, attention, and memory in the short term, and maybe over long-term use. So it seems likely to me that marijuana didn't help his grades.

Jason nods. "Yeah, I was worried about that, but, honestly, it seemed to help."

I'm thinking this information will not overjoy most school principals or college deans.

"Partly it's less nausea. You can't really pay attention to anything else when you've got that to deal with, but it was also the mental effects of the cancer treatment."

Jason's treatment regimen included high doses of corticosteroids such as prednisone, which can cause severe agitation, confusion, and bizarre behavior. When I was a resident, I was once called in the middle of the night to deal with a previously normal intern who'd dosed himself with prednisone for an uncomfortable poison ivy rash and was now taking his clothes off in the hospital's lobby.

That never happened to Jason. And although the nausea made it almost impossible for him to pay attention during three-hour classes, a few puffs on a vape pen actually helped him to calm down and focus. Surprisingly, he says it also helped his memory.

Now Jason is on a consolidation chemotherapy regimen that involves a week of drugs, followed by three weeks off. So does he keep using marijuana all the time?

Jason nods, like this is something he's thought about carefully.

"The first time, I just stopped it. Just cut it off. I finished the chemo on a Friday morning, and I used enough to get me through the weekend, then ended it. Makes sense, right?"

Not necessarily. I explain that some chemo causes nausea that can last for a week or more.

"Exactly. That's what I learned the hard way. It's not an on/off thing. I felt like crap the first couple of days. No one told me what to do or how to use it, you know? This stuff doesn't come with an instruction manual or one of those package inserts, but I got it figured out. I usually back off on the joints after a couple of days and get by on the vape pen. By the end of the month, I'm hardly using at all."

Jason thinks that's good. "I like being 'clean' for a little while. It makes me feel like I'm really healthy. Sure, I can use marijuana and make the people I hang out with *think* I'm healthy, but it's even more of a rush to be able to do that and be off all my drugs."

Where is he right now?

He smiles. "Right now I don't need anything. Haven't used in the last three days. I'll start again on Monday, but for now, I'm just a regular guy, and the nurses still say I look fabulous."

The Science of Nausea

It's likely that marijuana is effective in treating nausea. In fact, the evidence is probably better for nausea than it is for most other symptoms.

There are dozens of studies dating back to the 1950s that highlight the effect of marijuana and its related compounds on nausea. Not all of them are conclusive, but the weight of the evidence is pretty clearly on marijuana's side.[11] There's also a synthetic cannabinoid called nabilone that was developed in the 1970s to treat nausea related to chemotherapy, and it worked very well.[12]

How marijuana reduces nausea is a puzzle. The sensation of nausea is caused by the brain stem, the lower part of the brain that's responsible for basic functions like breathing and throwing up. However, there don't seem to be any cannabinoid receptors in the brain stem.

We know this because of a fascinating study in which researchers used twenty-two brains taken from three humans (who had died of non-neurologic disorders), twelve rats, four guinea pigs, two beagles, and one rhesus monkey. They sliced the brains paper thin, marinated those slices with a protein that binds to cannabinoid receptors, and linked that protein to a radioactive isotope. Then, they laid the slices of brain on a piece of radiation-sensitive film. Voilà: a map of the brain's cannabinoid receptors.[13]

The main result was that although these cannabinoid receptors are widely distributed in the brain, they don't seem to be located in the brain stem. If marijuana works to relieve nausea, it probably acts somewhere else—but where?

One possibility is the serotonin-based neural pathway in the gastrointestinal tract that involves the splenic nerve, which is one of the main nerves that controls digestion. The nausea caused by many chemotherapy agents seems to work through this pathway and, as we've seen, CBD binds to serotonin receptors. So, it's possible that the CBD in marijuana works in the same way that other widely prescribed drugs such as ondansetron work.

A second "vestibular" pathway seems to operate through the labyrinth system in the ear. When that system senses motion that's out of sync with what our eyes are seeing, we feel nauseated. If you've ever been car sick—or if you've had one too many martinis—you can thank that pathway. That pathway is different than the pathway by which chemotherapy drugs cause nausea, with different nerves, and different receptors. So we don't know whether marijuana is useful in treating nausea associated with car sickness.

Finally, there's an area of the brain that can make us feel nauseated. This area sits at the edge of the fourth ventricle, which is a sac that is filled with spinal fluid. It's called the "chemotrigger zone" because it acts as the body's poison control center. When it senses chemicals in spinal fluid that shouldn't be in us, it prompts us to vomit. As solutions go, it's not very elegant, but it's effective. Here, too, we don't know whether marijuana works on this pathway, but it's possible.

Even if marijuana is effective in treating nausea—and it seems to be—it probably doesn't work any better than standard drugs like lorazepam and prochlorperazine. At least, that's the impression I've gotten from several randomized controlled trials and reviews that have compared many of these drugs. And it may not work as well as drugs like ondansetron, one of the newer nausea drugs. However, not surprisingly, researchers who conducted an analysis of patient preferences that pooled eighteen studies found that three out of four patients preferred marijuana to other drugs.

Most of the studies of cannabinoids and nausea have used THC (dronabinol) or synthetics like nabilone, which are taken by mouth. There haven't been many studies of whole-plant marijuana and, as we've seen, natural marijuana has many cannabinoids, including CBD. At least some of those might relieve nausea, but you can only get them by using natural marijuana, or a mix like Sativex. There also haven't been many studies of smoked marijuana, which is important because we know that cannabinoids are at least twice as likely to get into the bloodstream if smoked than if they're taken by mouth. There's one study of smoked marijuana, though, that's interesting because it's a little unusual.

Instead of studying patients receiving chemotherapy, researchers used ipecac to make people nauseated. Ipecac causes nausea and vomiting by inducing the gastrointestinal tract to release serotonin, just as some chemotherapy drugs do, so it's used as a way to test potential treatments for the sort of chemotherapy-induced nausea that Jason experienced. The study found that smoked marijuana was more effective than placebo marijuana in reducing nausea and vomiting.[14] ("Placebo marijuana" is marijuana from which THC and CBD have been removed, in much the same way that caffeine is removed from coffee beans to make decaf.) However, it was less effective than ondansetron, which is the drug that's most commonly used for chemotherapy-related nausea.

Overall, even though we're not sure how marijuana controls nausea, I'm pretty convinced that it does. Particularly nausea that's a side effect of chemotherapy, and possibly nausea due to other causes. We also know that there are cannabinoid receptors in the gastrointestinal pathway, a key mechanism for nausea. So Jason was probably on the right track.

The Man Who Pretended to Eat

Many people with serious illnesses like cancer or AIDS lose weight for reasons that have nothing to do with nausea. How this cachexia, or wasting syndrome of weight loss and muscle atrophy, happens isn't well understood, but it's likely a combination of decreased appetite and increased metabolism that burns calories at an accelerated rate. The result is that people don't eat enough to keep pace, and they lose weight.

Some of my patients with cancer joke that this might be a good thing, but it's not. Most of us could afford to lose a little fat, but the weight loss of diseases like cancer and AIDS takes far too much. More important, it also takes muscle. So people with cachexia often lose muscle strength, and they feel weak and tired. That's what happened to Joseph.

Joseph tells me he's in his late sixties, but his hollow cheeks and prominent cheekbones make him look much, much older. His most striking feature, though, are bright blue eyes that peek out under a white shock of hair that curtains his forehead.

He's probably the oldest medical marijuana patient I've met. At least, he's the oldest person I know is a patient. And he's using medical marijuana to stimulate his appetite, which is one of its oldest medical uses.

Joseph says his lung cancer was diagnosed about a year ago. Cure wasn't possible, so Joseph only agreed to take chemotherapy drugs that wouldn't cause serious side effects, and that he could take as a pill. Things went well for a while, and he even felt better.

"But then I started losing weight. A lot of weight. At least fifty or sixty pounds just evaporated."

He didn't feel like eating, but he *wanted* to. Especially when his kids and grandchildren were visiting. He wanted to be part of the family, and that meant joining in meals.

"We've got an enormous Italian family, and meals are a big deal. They're sacred. Showing up and not eating . . . well, that's just wrong. So I would pretend to eat. Just sort of push food around on my plate and make a big show of taking every bite."

When his son-in-law suggested marijuana, Joseph decided to give it a try. After some trial and error, he started using little marijuana-infused pieces of chocolate. Now he has one after every meal, and he's found that he usually has an appetite before the next meal comes around, and he's also sleeping better at night.

"I've just been more of a nice guy all around."

I laugh, a little uncertainly.

"No, seriously. I mean, I was never a nasty guy. I'm lucky I've got a good family, and we're close. But this cancer tries your patience, you know?"

I remember that Caleb, the blacksmith I introduced you to in chapter 1, told me something similar. He wasn't talking about using marijuana recreationally, but rather because it toned down some of the anger he felt over dying of cancer in his forties. I wonder whether Joseph would use marijuana for the same reason.

He smiles.

"Well, when you say it like that, I might not. I mean, that's something that people ought to be able to work out on their own, you know?" He pauses. "But yeah. I just might."

How Hunger Works

Although there's pretty good evidence for the use of cannabinoids to treat nausea, the evidence for appetite and weight gain is surprisingly mixed. That's surprising because it's been used for this purpose for a long time, and because everyone knows that marijuana gives you the munchies.

In order to understand how marijuana might help Joseph gain weight, it helps to think of appetite and weight gain as two separate issues. Usually if you're hungry, you eat, and if you eat, you gain weight. But it seems as though marijuana and its constituent parts are much more likely to increase appetite than they are to increase weight.

One of the earliest studies of marijuana and appetite was conducted in a locked ward. Specifically, a "residential laboratory designed for continuous observation of human behavior over extended periods."[15] In this case, an "extended period" was thirteen days. Subjects were given access to marijuana joints, or placebo joints, and were monitored very carefully. Their snacks were weighed, and their wrappers and leftovers were scrutinized. "No communication outside of the laboratory was permitted," the report says.

After almost two weeks of weighing and measuring, researchers found that these subjects increased their food intake by roughly 20 percent, and that increase was due to snacking between meals. Meal consumption actually decreased a little.

Subsequent studies have confirmed that both marijuana and dronabinol (THC) increase appetite,[16] but how that happens is a bit of a mystery.

One guess is that THC acts on CB1 receptors in the hypothalamus, but it's probably much more complicated.

We know that THC affects some of the hormones that are involved in regulating appetite. One study let seven HIV-positive men smoke either marijuana or placebo marijuana, and then measured several hormones.[17] What was most interesting about that study was that the researchers didn't find any effect on the best-known metabolic hormone, insulin.

However, they did find that marijuana increased ghrelin, a hormone that promotes appetite. It also decreased a hormone called peptide YY, which is normally higher after a meal and causes us to feel full. The researchers also measured marijuana's influence on leptin, whose effects are more complicated. It seems to undergo hardwired changes through a twenty-four-hour cycle (highest at night), but it's also reduced after meals. In this study, marijuana also decreased leptin levels.

Of the hormones I've mentioned, only leptin seemed to mirror THC blood levels. Graphs of THC versus the other hormones just look like a series of random dots, which suggests that if something in marijuana is influencing those hormones, it must be another cannabinoid, like CBD. So as we've seen before in studies of pain and anxiety, THC may be less important than we thought, and the humble CBD molecule, or another cannabinoid, might be more useful.

Even if we don't know yet how marijuana increases appetite, it's pretty clear that it does. But appetite doesn't help if a cancer patient like Joseph isn't regaining the weight he's lost. Can marijuana help with that, too?

In general, clinical trials have been disappointing. The evidence for weight gain is pretty limited in AIDS,[18] and the evidence in patients with cancer isn't much better.[19] These trials have found that appetite does increase, and people eat more. But they don't eat enough to keep pace with the revved-up metabolism that these diseases cause.

One exception, sort of, is a study in which some patients with AIDS got dronabinol. Those patients did not gain weight, but the patients in the placebo group lost weight.[20] That may seem like dronabinol won on a technicality, but remember that Joseph lost fifty or sixty pounds in a couple of months. In conditions like cancer or AIDS, which can cause profound weight loss, sometimes just holding steady is actually a victory.

Even though marijuana probably doesn't help people gain weight, it does increase appetite, and that's important. If your family sits down to dinner every night, eating means you get to participate. And that's worth something to Joseph and other patients.

The Woman Who Healed Herself

It's plausible that marijuana could treat insomnia or seizures or nausea, because these problems all have links to the brain, and we know that the brain has a lot of cannabinoid receptors. But there are other uses that are still theoretical, like treating cancer. The idea might seem bizarre, yet there are many people who are pinning all of their hopes on marijuana rather than proven chemotherapy.

Are those hopes rational? I'm skeptical. It's one thing to suggest that the cannabinoids in marijuana might bind to receptors in the short term to relieve a symptom like nausea or pain, because we know that those receptors and pathways exist. And if it's not effective, people will figure that out pretty quickly.

On the other hand, it's hard to see how marijuana might cure cancer. Besides, putting your hopes on marijuana to cure cancer is—quite literally—a life-and-death decision that I'd be very reluctant to make. But I've met one woman who has made that decision, and she's convinced that marijuana is saving her life.

Sheila is a slight woman in her fifties, with short, spiky blond hair. When we met in a café in a hip Denver neighborhood, Sheila wanted very much to tell her story. About a year ago she was diagnosed with diffuse large-cell lymphoma, which is very aggressive and fast growing. Sheila's oncologist told her that she had a 60 percent chance of a cure, but she struggled through the first round of chemotherapy.

"I got through most of it," she says. She pauses. "Well, some of it, anyway."

She lived alone, and found it hard to take care of herself when the chemotherapy made her weak and tired. Even getting to clinic appointments was difficult, and she often forgot to take her medications. So when Sheila heard about an "easy" cure, she figured she'd look into it.

What she found was hash oil like the kind Cal and Cindy got for their daughter Randi. The oil that Sheila used was being promoted as a cure-all for many types of cancer, and at the heart of that promotional effort was a man named Rick Simpson, a Canadian who is convinced that hash oil is the cure for all manner of ills, from arthritis to cancer.

Simpson has found adherents. Lots of them. Many people like Sheila have accepted his advice and put their lives into his hands. They've followed his instructions and put their trust in cannabis oil to treat anything from relatively benign and slow-growing skin cancers to very aggressive malignancies like Sheila's.

In a profile written for *High Times* magazine, Rick Simpson sounds like an evangelist driven by faith.[21] His oil has wrought cures that are described as "miraculous," and he's quoted as claiming a success rate of 70 percent with patients who were thought to be dying. Simpson's story has become a legend of sorts in the marijuana community, so it's difficult to separate fact from fiction, but the key points are that Simpson's cousin died a very difficult and painful death from cancer in 1972. Two years later, Simpson heard a news report about a study that had found that THC reduced the size of tumors in mice.

The idea of using cannabinoids sat in the back of Simpson's mind for almost thirty years, until 2001. After a workplace accident, he decided to start making and using cannabinoid-rich oil to treat himself for tinnitus (ringing in his ears), memory loss, and other problems. The oil worked so well that when his doctor told him three spots on his skin were cancer, he tried painting them with the oil he'd been using. One, on his face, was surgically removed, but he treated the two remaining spots and they disappeared. A few months later, the lesion that had been surgically removed recurred. Simpson treated it in the same way and it, too, vanished.

It was at that point that he became the evangelist he's known as today. First, he treated his mother's psoriasis, and then he treated dozens of people for various skin conditions. According to legend, all of those supplicants were cured. And even a cursory Internet search turns up testimonials of patients whose cancers were controlled, or reduced, or even cured by using the kind of concentrated cannabinoid oil that Simpson promoted.

Word got out through Simpson's speaking engagements, information on his website, and, of course, word of mouth. However, from what I've been able to learn, he never sold the oil that he made. Initially he produced it and gave it away. In later years he used marijuana given to him by farmers, returning some oil to the farmers and giving the rest away. Whatever his motives, profit didn't seem to be one of them.

The doses that patients use are rather high. An often-cited figure is 60 grams of oil for a full treatment, typically in doses of a gram (1,000 milligrams) a day. So if this oil has a THC concentration of, say, 50 percent, people would be taking 500 milligrams a day. Typical doses of THC taken by mouth are less than 50 milligrams, so that's a whopping dose.

However, Simpson has said he prefers hash oil made from *indica* strains of marijuana, which tend to be low in THC and high in CBD. And as Cal and Cindy discovered, some *indica*-derived oils don't have any THC at all. So although 500 milligrams of THC would probably make people very stoned and anxious, a gram of oil that contains 50 percent CBD (500 milligrams) would be lower than what was used in the studies of CBD and anxiety I described earlier (up to 600 milligrams).

That's in theory. In reality, most plants—and therefore the oils that are made from them—do contain THC and CBD. Cal and Cindy got their oil tested before they gave it to Randi, but most people aren't so careful, so Simpson's oil almost certainly contains some THC, and probably has at least some psychoactive effects.

Word of Rick Simpson's success has spread, and his oil is credited with miraculous cures of everything from diabetes to advanced lung cancer. Those paeans drew the attention of the Royal Canadian Mounted Police, who repeatedly raided Simpson's home and on one productive visit in 2005 reportedly seized 1,620 marijuana plants.

Now Simpson is making himself scarce, and there are reports that he's living overseas. I'm not sure whether he's still supplying his oil to patients, but he's keeping a lower profile. Nevertheless, he has so many disciples preaching the gospel of oil that his movement has enough momentum to continue without him.

Sheila started using the oil alongside her chemotherapy at first, but soon she stopped the chemotherapy altogether. She tells me she's been on nothing but the oil for about seven months now.

She's brought a stack of CT scans with her, and each is flagged with a dated Post-it Note. They were all taken using the dye that highlights abnormal tissue like cancer, so lymphoma and enlarged lymph nodes show up as bright white.

The first scan Sheila shows me was done in March 2013. It's a series of cross-sectional images of her chest, arranged from top to bottom. I'm not a radiologist, but even I can see abnormal images in the mediastinum—the region around the heart and between the left and right lungs. It looks as though there's a large mass there that's maybe six by eight centimeters. I also see scattered bright spots that are enlarged lymph nodes where her cancer has spread. Maybe there are other abnormalities, but already I can see more than enough to terrify most people, and this was the scan that Sheila got when she was diagnosed.

Next she shows me a scan from early June 2013, which looks like it might have come from a different person. At first I think that her lymphoma is completely gone, but there's still some swelling in the mediastinum. Just a little. I can barely make out a mass that's not much bigger than a walnut.

The last scan is dated October 2013, and it looks identical to the one done in June. Even putting them side by side, I can't tell the difference. In fact, I check the dates on the scans themselves to make sure that Sheila's labels are truthful. They are.

"You see?"

I do. Diffuse B-cell lymphoma can be aggressive and fast growing, so the absence of any progression, at least based on the scans in front of me, is surprising. Diffuse B-cell lymphoma typically responds quickly to chemotherapy, so lymphoma might have shrunk because of the treatment she got, but her scans have been stable for four months with no treatment other than the oil that she was using.

"That's proof, isn't it?" Sheila asks me. "I can't understand why people don't see this. Why don't they understand that this is the cure everyone's been looking for? And it's right here." She pauses and shakes her head so vigorously that her earrings swing in wide, agitated arcs.

"If people would just wake up," she says. "So many people could benefit. Without all of the misery of chemotherapy."

I think it's safe to say I'm impressed, but I'm a long way from being convinced, and one story is hardly proof.

There's a lot about Sheila's story that we don't know. For instance, we don't know how much chemotherapy she received. In fact, if you don't trust my reading of that CT scan—and you probably shouldn't—Sheila's experience may be nothing more than a lucky, long-lasting remission (reduction in tumor size) induced by chemotherapy.

If Sheila's right, that's great. But what if she's not? She's betting her life on a few drops of oil, and if she's wrong she could die. The same is true of all the people whose stories I've read online, claiming that Simpson's oil cured their lung cancer or breast cancer or melanoma. No one knows how many people are trusting Simpson's oil, but there are probably a lot of lives at risk.

So, I set out in search of someone who can give me the big picture of what marijuana is good for and what it isn't. If Raphael Mechoulam is the dignified grandfather of medical marijuana, then Donald Abrams is its kindly, slightly radical uncle. The kind of guy everyone hopes will show up at Thanksgiving dinner to liven things up. He's one of the most respected voices in favor of medical marijuana, and something of an iconoclast, but he's also an oncologist. I figure if anyone can give me a balanced view of whether marijuana can cure cancer, it's him.

Miracle Cures and Mistakes

Donald Abrams is not an easy man to find. In fact, I wander around San Francisco General Hospital for an hour before I wash up on the grounds of a structure that's known somewhat ominously as Building 80.

Abrams looks disappointingly normal. He has a pleasant, open face that reminds me more than a little of Mr. Rogers. Conservatively dressed in a blue button-down oxford, gray flannel trousers, and sober tie, his square glasses and short silver-gray hair make him look like an investment banker.

Any doubts that I'm the right place are assuaged by his desk, a cheerful melee of patient charts and medical journals. That scholarly stuff is happily interspersed with a large and diverse collection of jade statues, vases, and enough Chinese teas to open a modest tearoom.

So . . . can marijuana treat cancer?

Abrams shakes his head in what looks like despair. I'm thinking that's my answer right there.

"It really hurts me when patients come to me wanting to treat their cancer," he says. "Marijuana can do a lot, but that . . ." He shakes his head again.

What about Rick Simpson's claims?

He nods. "He's on the lam now. No one knows where he is."

So the promise of a cancer cure is just wishful thinking?

"Whether it cures malignancies, we don't know."

I'm guessing that he's not optimistic. Later, we talk about marijuana's benefits for a variety of symptoms, and he's generally enthusiastic. He acknowledges a lack of good evidence, but he's still optimistic about the ability of marijuana to relieve symptoms. Not for treating cancer, though.

So how do these myths gain traction? Is it just what people want to believe?

That's a lot of it, Abrams admits, but it's more complicated. He points out that the definition of a "cure" in the oncology world is five years of disease-free survival. That's five years during which there's no evidence of cancer, after which it's usually safe to say that it's really gone. So if Sheila's lymphoma disappears and stays gone for five years, she could count that as a cure, but if it's only been gone for a few months, there's a good chance that it will come back.

That five-year definition is important, Abrams says, because the highly concentrated oil she used hasn't been legally available for very long. Many people, like Sheila, have used it in the last few years. It's just too soon to say that any of them are cured.

Regardless, Sheila isn't even "disease free." I saw clear evidence of swollen lymph nodes on her CT scan. I'm betting those abnormal lymphoma cells are still there, waiting to start growing again.

Abrams also reminds me that many types of cancer don't grow steadily. They stop and start, and sometimes seem to shrink spontaneously. He suspects that many stories of "cures" might be cancers that tend to shrink spontaneously, and he tells me about his own experience with that phenomenon.

"I have a basal cell on my chest that I can say comes and goes." Abrams shrugs. "Every time I think about getting it removed, it's gone." He doesn't need to point out that if he were a marijuana user, it would be pretty likely, even inevitable, that he would convince himself that it was the marijuana that was responsible for that improvement.

Finally, there are challenges of accurate diagnosis and staging (a measure of how advanced a cancer is). If the initial diagnosis is incorrect, or if the stage is wrong, it's easy to convince yourself that what was really an error was the result of marijuana.

"I guess I've been party to that," he admits sheepishly.

He's referring to the case of Michelle Aldrich. She and her husband, Michael, are staunch advocates for the legalization of medical marijuana and friends of Abrams's. When Michelle was diagnosed with non-small-cell lung cancer in January of 2012, she turned quickly to marijuana.

"She got chemotherapy, and also used cannabis oil. Then when she went to surgery in May of 2012, they couldn't find any evidence of disease. None, and that's unusual. So that's what I said to her. Not a miracle, but close." In March of 2013, her CT scan was clear.

Although that sounds impressive, I'm anticipating a "but."

"I thought she had stage IIIB cancer, but she really had stage IIIA. It's not much of a difference, but it's enough."

Stage IIIB cancer has spread to lymph nodes on the other side of the chest, but stage IIIA hasn't. That spread is bad news, because it makes IIIB cancer much harder to treat than IIIA. For a patient like Michelle with stage IIIA cancer to have a 50 percent reduction in tumor after chemotherapy isn't unheard of, and for her to be apparently disease free after surgery is at least possible.

So are Sheila, Michelle, and all of Rick Simpson's disciples simply deluded? That's a tough question for someone like Abrams. He's an advocate of medical marijuana, but he's also a buttoned-down oncologist. However much he argues for integrative therapy and holistic healing, he also pushes chemo.

Abrams tells me there's a lot of evidence from cell culture experiments indicating that marijuana's cannabinoids might slow the growth of cancer. These are experiments in which tumor cells are grown in a laboratory as bacteria are cultured in a petri dish. Then cannabinoids are added, and their effects on cell growth are measured. Ideally, you'd want to see those cells stop growing and dividing.

Remember that back in the 1970s, Rick Simpson heard a news report about THC reducing the size of brain tumors in mice. That wasn't science fiction. In fact, Abrams tells me, it's known that cannabinoids can slow the growth of lung cancer tumor cells, but because of prejudices against marijuana, and difficulties in procuring it legally for research purposes, the results of those initial studies funded by the U.S. National Cancer Institute just sat there, unexplored.

Now, though, researchers are starting to make up for lost time. Some recent studies have confirmed the antitumor effects of natural and synthetic cannabinoids. Other studies have shown that cannabinoids injected into mice with tumors can cause those tumors to shrink, and the same effects seem to be true across a wide range of tumor types, including tumors of the lung, breast, colon, thyroid, pancreas, as well as melanoma and lymphoma, just to name a few.

One interesting result of these studies is that cannabinoids seem to spare normal cells. Many of the well-known and unpleasant side effects of chemotherapy and radiation therapy, such as anemia, low white blood cell count, hair loss, and diarrhea, are the result of collateral damage to normal cells. If we can avoid that damage, cancer treatment would be much more tolerable.

Cannabinoids also seem to slow the abnormal formation of new blood vessels in tumors. This so-called angiogenesis is what makes it possible for tumors to grow and spread. It works in much the same way that freeways promote faster transportation and let a city expand quickly out into suburbs. Cannabinoids block those new blood vessels, possibly by reducing concentrations of vascular endothelial growth factor (VEGF), a local hormone that is needed for the formation of new blood vessels.

The effect is like slapping a lot of regulations and zoning restrictions on construction businesses, with the result that highways become hard to build. No highways, no suburbs. No new blood vessels, no cancer growth.

Abrams says that THC might also block the effects of epidermal growth factor on cells' ability to grow and migrate, possibly making tumor cells less invasive. Experiments in mice have found that another cannabinoid, cannabigerol (CBG), slows the growth of cancer cells.[22] As with CBD, CBG doesn't seem to have any psychoactive effects, and it probably works through receptors other than CB1 and CB2.

There are probably also other mechanisms we haven't begun to understand. Abrams mentions a protein known as Id-1. It's one of many proteins thought to be responsible for controlling the rate at which cells proliferate, and Abrams says that CBD has been shown to reduce the production of Id-1 in breast cancer cells.[23]

Most of Abrams's mini-lecture is over my head, and I get the sense that this science is changing at a rapid pace. It's bewildering in a good way, though. Now I can see why people like Sheila are so excited, and at least there's some real science here.

But there isn't enough science to pin all of our hopes on. Imagine if, on their first flight, Orville and Wilbur Wright had aimed the Wright Flyer toward France. The theory was sound, and flight was possible, so why not?

That's pretty much what Rick Simpson's acolytes are doing. People like Sheila who forgo chemotherapy for marijuana are turning their backs on something with known benefits for what is—at least right now—a forlorn hope. That is, until science catches up.

Abrams thinks it's possible that that might happen someday.

"If it's going to work anywhere," he says, "the brain would be a good place to start." He'd like to do a study of hash oil on a rare but horribly aggressive form of brain tumor called a glioblastoma multiforme (GBM). It's difficult to treat, and almost impossible to cure. It tends to affect younger patients, which makes it particularly scary, but there's reason for optimism, Abrams says, because of one small study that was done in Spain.[24]

That study enrolled nine patients with recurrent glioblastoma, all of whom had a dismal prognosis. They underwent surgery to cut away some of the tumor, and then a catheter was placed with its tip in the center of what remained. Then the researchers injected concentrated THC (96.5 percent) through the skull, directly into the tumor. The injections were safe, and—surprisingly—didn't seem to produce any psychoactive effects. Because the researchers had excised some tumor cells from the surgery, they were able to culture those cells and then to determine that THC slowed their growth.

Abrams explains that the oil he wants to test would need to be reviewed by the Food and Drug Administration as a new molecular entity (NME). (The irony that this acronym, NME, sounds like "enemy" is not lost on medical marijuana proponents.) That's an enormous problem because in order to obtain FDA approval, Abrams would need to prove that marijuana oil is safe in animals, and that would require time and research funding that he doesn't have.

Abrams notes that he's had some success in convincing regulators that CBD doesn't need an NME. Now he's using CBD in a study he's doing that enrolls patients with sickle cell anemia. It's been long, hard work, involving testimonials from researchers and even pictures of dispensary signs advertising marijuana that is high in CBD.

I ask Abrams where the field of medical marijuana research is going next.

Up until now, Abrams has been the genial host, but something I've said seems to rub him the wrong way. He's still polite, but he seems frustrated, too.

"When you say 'field' I'm not sure what you mean. You know there aren't many of us doing this research."

I protest that I'm sure that there will be more researchers as marijuana gains acceptance. If more people are using it for medical purposes, we'll need more data to tell us how it works, but he's not convinced.

One problem with my naïveté, he points out, is funding. How do you fund research on a plant? Companies can make synthetics, like dronabinol, or they can create proprietary mixtures of natural extracts, like Sativex, but if you want to study a plant that doesn't have a patent, and which a company can't make money on, then you need to turn to public funding. Abrams knows it's not a promising strategy to turn to the National Institutes of Health, including the National Cancer Institute.

Grant reviews are notoriously slow to catch up with science. As a palliative care researcher, it's taken me a while to convince funders that research that makes people more comfortable is as important as research that helps people live longer, but we're making progress.

That's only one part of the problem, Abrams says. The larger issue, and the one that has him frustrated, is his concern that even if he and the rest of the "field" do good research, those results won't change policy.

"There are some people who think that science drives the train. That science guides what's prescribed, and what's allowed."

I admit that I'm one of those people, but Abrams isn't.

"Any drug that makes you feel good has a black mark against it. And that's true no matter how effective a drug might be."

Other countries, such as Canada, have moved ahead in making marijuana more available.

"A few countries have taken bold steps, and haven't disappeared from the face of the earth. That's true." But he's not optimistic; he doesn't see a future in which marijuana is widely available as a medicine.

A Wonder Drug?

I'll admit that marijuana seems to offer more benefits than I imagined it would, though it's by no means a wonder drug. The most we can say right now with any confidence is that it probably works for some symptoms.

It seems to be effective for neuropathic pain, which is impressive because neuropathic pain seems to be so resistant to medical treatment. Although the evidence for treating regular, so-called nociceptive pain is weak, I think we might begin to see that evidence eventually. I'm particularly optimistic about that possibility because regular pain is due in part to inflammation, which is caused by white blood cells. So I'm hopeful that there might be a way to exploit CBD's effects on those white blood cells to treat regular pain, too.

We already have a lot of evidence that marijuana is effective in treating nausea. I'm particularly pleased by that conclusion, because when nausea is difficult to treat, I often find myself at a loss. Severe nausea can be so disruptive that it can ruin my patients' quality of life, just as it did to Jason, the young man who looked fabulous on chemo. So, even if marijuana isn't more effective than other treatments are, having one more option is good news.

I'm less enthusiastic about evidence that marijuana increases appetite. True, the evidence is there, and I'm convinced it does induce people to eat more, but that just isn't something that bothers my patients very much. Still, for those people like Joseph for whom meals are family affairs, marijuana is worth a try.

Finally, even if we agree that concentrated marijuana oil isn't a substitute for chemotherapy—and it isn't—there's a lot of research here to be excited about. For instance, there's pretty persuasive evidence that cannabinoids like THC can slow tumor growth and prevent cancer spread, at least in the laboratory. So, although it's premature to put all of your hopes on Rick Simpson's oil, as Sheila did, it's possible that someday marijuana might produce treatments that really do work.

Sheila died of her lymphoma in March 2015. She did resume chemotherapy in the last months of her life, but by that time her lymphoma had spread too widely and was no longer curable.

4

Beer and Brownies

It's a beautiful, warm spring afternoon, and I'm sitting in a pretty walled garden sipping tea with a friend. Lisa's German shepherd is lounging at my feet, and there is a plateful of fresh chocolate chip cookies within easy reach. What could be better?

Well, this day could be a little better—at least in some ways—if I were stoned. But I'm not. Not at all.

And that's disappointing, because I was hoping to get just a little high this afternoon. The "tea" that Lisa prepared shortly after I arrived isn't really tea. It's actually made from part of a dried marijuana bud that has been steeped in almost-boiling water for precisely eight minutes. The resulting liquid was then poured into a chipped enamel mug. I drank it, along with a refill, with no appreciable effects whatsoever. Except for a rather full bladder, I regret to report that this marijuana tea has done absolutely nothing for me.

That's too bad, because I'm interested in finding new and different ways to get the active ingredients of marijuana into people. Sure, you can light up a joint. The marijuana burns, and the THC and CBD are vaporized, and you inhale them.

But there are many reasons why you might not want to light up a joint. For instance, the smell of marijuana smoke is unmistakable, and it's virtually impossible to smoke a joint discreetly, surreptitiously in a public place. If you're afraid of what other people might think of you, and especially if you're worried about the legality of public marijuana use, then you'll have to limit your smoking to the privacy of your own home.

Even there, you might not want your friends or family to know what you're using, or how often you're using it. And you might be worried about exposing other people to secondhand smoke. Finally, if you have lung problems such as emphysema or asthma, smoking a joint is a bad idea. I think it's safe to say that almost all of the medical marijuana users I've met so far would like to have a way of using it, at least on some occasions, that is not as obvious as lighting up a joint.

Are there other options? There are, and we've seen a few of them already. Joseph in chapter 3 ate marijuana-infused pieces of chocolate, and there's also the oil that Randi and Sheila used. And the marijuana tea that I just sampled.

However, as I just discovered, these options are not equally effective. Some offer a great way to get the active ingredients of marijuana into people, but others work less well. And others are just a waste of time (and marijuana).

While the previous two chapters were an introduction to what marijuana can do for us, this chapter is more of a practical cookbook for its use. I'll introduce you to marijuana ointment, beer, and wine. I'll tell you what we know about how these various methods of ingestion affect people, and whether they have the medical effects that we want them to have. But first we need to understand where THC and CBD come from, and for that I need to introduce you to a marijuana plant.

That's *Ms. Sativa* to You

I'm about to meet an example of *Cannabis sativa*, and I'm excited. After a year of research about its medical effects, I finally get to see where marijuana comes from, up close and personal.

A fellow named Roger will be making this introduction, and he knows his way around marijuana plants. He also knows his way around the law, which is decidedly not on his side. Roger lives in a state where medical marijuana is legal. However, he provides his product to friends and acquaintances for free, or in exchange for a modest donation. He isn't a licensed grower and isn't protected by the laws that exist. That's why I've agreed not to mention where he lives, or where he grows what he grows.

Roger is a middle-aged, heavyset, avuncular guy who speaks slowly and walks with a cane. He's vague about his medical history but mentions that he has "a couple of chronic conditions," at least one of which led him to begin experimenting with marijuana for his personal use more than a decade ago. This is a common theme. Many of the people I've met in the marijuana business began using it to treat their own medical problems and later joined the vanguard of activists, growers, and purveyors.

Roger and I are in an improvised greenhouse on the top floor of his house. One room has been converted into a space that's about fifteen feet square, with bay windows on two adjacent sides and a row of skylights overhead. The room is bright, warm, and humid, with a dense scent of humus and peat and overripe fruit.

The plants I'm here to meet are arrayed neatly in three ranks on low benches constructed of rough planks resting on cinder blocks. There are perhaps twenty of them, each in one-gallon pots. I expected more, but Roger explains that you can't pack the plants in too tightly. They need airflow. (Actually, "breathing room" is the phrase he uses to describe these plants that, in a few short weeks, are going to go up in smoke.)

Roger explains that there are two principal strains of the *Cannabis* plant: *sativa* and *indica*. *Sativa* strains emphasize psychoactive THC over CBD. On the other hand, the *indica* strains that Rick Simpson uses to make his oil have more CBD and less THC. And, as Cal and Cindy discovered, some *indica* strains are almost entirely CBD. So *sativa* strains tend to be more popular among recreational users, whereas medical marijuana users tend to use both *sativa* and *indica*, and sometimes a mixture. However, it's impossible to tell them apart just by looking at them, because there's so much variation in physical appearance among strains within each species. Some strains are tall and thin, while others are short and squat. And their THC and CBD concentrations vary, too.

It's like the differences among dogs, Roger explains. Just as dachshunds and Great Danes are all *Canis familiaris*, vastly different-looking plants can be grouped under either *sativa* or *indica*.

There is some debate about this, actually. Another group, *ruderalis*, has been proposed as a third species, but current theory favors two, although there's a dissenting group that argues for one overarching species that includes all cannabis plants.

Roger guides me down the alley that separates two of the benches, his slippers rustling on the clear plastic beneath our feet. Along the way, he explains what I'm seeing on either side of me.

"Here you've got a perfect example. Just starting to bud."

We stop in front of a plant that's about two feet tall. It has a long, central stem with a fringe of thin, serrated leaves at the top. And all along the stem, lower down, are smaller, less-developed pinwheels of leaves.

It's immediately recognizable as a marijuana plant, at least to me, because I've just finished reading the official U.S. government field guide to pot, *Marihuana: Its Identification*. This handy reference was published in 1938 by no less an authority than the U.S. Bureau of Narcotics. It's a bit dated, perhaps. Then again, not much has really changed in the science of marijuana's identification.

But for those of you who haven't read this manual, here's a quick summary. Typical cannabis plants have groups of seven symmetrical, serrated leaves that you can think of as being arranged around an imaginary clock face. There's a long leaf at 12:00, and two smaller leaves at 11:00 and 1:00. There are two more at 9:00 and 3:00, and two more stunted leaves at about 7:00 and 5:00.

"To the experienced observer the appearance of the hemp plant," the field guide promises, "marihuana (*Cannabis sativa*), is as distinctive as is the appearance of corn or wheat to the farmer."

Marijuana's most distinctive feature, though, which I've never seen on an ear of corn or a sheaf of wheat, is its buds. They're where the action is. And they're the reason I'm here.

Most of these buds are still immature, Roger says. They're green, and about 1.5 inches wide. The buds on top of the plant are a little more well developed, and easily recognizable. The ones farther down on a plant are just beginning to form.

Roger points to a plant in front of us. This particular plant is a *Cannabis sativa* strain known as Key Lime Kush, in the same way that a dog (*Canis familiaris*) could be classified as a dachshund or a boxer. And just as those breeds have recognizable characteristics, marijuana strains have both physical traits (e.g., size, shape) and typical ratios of THC to CBD.

He explains that some buds have stamens (the male plants) and others have pistils (the female plants). Many plants will have either male or female buds, but sometimes a plant will have both. "Some people see that, and they claim that cannabis is a hermaphrodite," says Roger. From under his bushy eyebrows he looks at me closely. I assure him that I have never claimed any such thing.

On any given plant, it's important to know the sex of a bud. Female buds are rich in trichomes, which are literally hairs. They're fuzzy bits that would look like tiny nail heads if you put them under the microscope. And trichomes are rich in THC and CBD. Male buds have fewer trichomes, and therefore much less THC and CBD. They also have a lot of seeds. So as soon as Roger starts seeing those stamens appear on a plant, he plucks those male buds off the plant and discards them. In marijuana husbandry, you really don't want to be a guy.

The U.S. Bureau of Narcotics is careful to point out the significance of trichomes, too. "No plant material which fails to show them can be marijuana."[1]

Actually, these trichomes are only rich in THC and CBD once they've been dried. In its natural state, a marijuana plant doesn't contain much THC or CBD. Instead, it has the acidic forms of those molecules, tetrahydrocannabinolic acid and cannabidiolic acid (known as THCA and CBDA). These molecules probably don't have much of an effect on our cannabinoid receptors. So a salad made of marijuana greens won't get you high. Instead, the buds need to be dried and heated to convert their cannabinoids to THC and CBD, which our bodies will recognize.

And flowers are pollinated by bees?

For this I get a look of dismay.

"No, cannabis is wind pollinated. You don't need insects or birds. Cannabis pollinates itself to produce flowers."

And when does that happen? Can he control when flowers appear?

Roger nods, and explains that *indica* and *sativa* are "short day plants." He can force them to flower by cutting back on the light they're exposed to.

Ruderalis plants—which are either a subgroup or a separate species of *Cannabis sativa*—have a different method of flowering. They're not triggered by light, but by time. Once plants reach a certain age, they begin to flower, regardless of the ambient light.

As we talk, Roger is checking his crop, looking for signs of rot or insects. He offers some other husbandry tips over his shoulder. Cannabis likes a constant temperature of between 75 and 80 degrees, he tells me. And not too much water.

And then, when they're ready, he harvests the buds?

He smiles. "Not just the buds. That's a common misconception. Actually you can harvest the whole plant. Look."

He plucks off a leaf and holds it up to a skylight. As I look up, I can see a fine white haze on the undersides of the leaf and the stem.

Trichomes?

Roger nods. He reminds me that THC and CBD are most concentrated in the trichomes, which are mostly in the buds. But they also appear on leaves, so he harvests everything. His customers smoke the buds or use them to make edibles, but they use other parts, too.

I'm curious—Roger keeps referring to the plants as cannabis. I ask why he doesn't call them marijuana plants.

He reminds me that "marijuana" (or, in the early twentieth century, "marihuana") is the name that its opponents bestowed on it to make it seem more foreign, and dangerous.

"The proper name," and here he stands a little straighter, "is *Canna-*

bis sativa." And, since we're really only interested in the female plants, I suppose the proper form of address would be Ms. Sativa.

This discussion about THC and CBD content makes me think of a question that I suspect would be of intense interest to any marijuana user. Can he control the amount of THC or CBD a plant produces?

Roger nods. "Through breeding, sure. It's pretty predictable, actually. Say you've got a drug plant and a nondrug plant."

Those terms are shorthand for describing plants that have high and low THC:CBD ratios, respectively. However, as we've seen, some researchers like Barth Wilsey think that we may have this backward, and that CBD might actually be a more effective "drug" than THC.

"If you breed them, your first generation is going to have a ratio that's in between. Kind of like . . ."

Breeding a boxer and a Great Dane?

Roger nods, pleased. He looks like he's making a mental note to recycle this analogy.

So how would you increase cannabinoid production?

Now Roger looks truly interested. It's the first of my questions that has seemed to wake him up. He smiles, and stops prodding the plant in front of him. Then he walks to the other end of the room, holding up a single forefinger. Wait.

He opens a low metal cabinet tucked under a window and pulls out a one-gallon plastic jug that's about half full of a dark brown liquid. He comes back over to me, opens the cap, and proffers it at nose height.

It smells sweet. And earthy. Like . . . molasses?

Roger nods. He explains that he mixes it with water and pours it onto each plant's roots. He's not sure how it increases a plant's THC, but he's pretty sure it does.

I suggest that he could try it on some of his plants but not others. Then get the buds tested for THC and CBD content. A randomized controlled trial.

Roger gets a faraway look. "You know, with the next crop, I just might. That testing is expensive, but hey—think of the contribution I could make."

The Fighting Mice Test

Roger is still thinking about his potential contribution to the science of cannabis husbandry as we make our way down the stairs. But I have one last question for him, which I ask over my shoulder.

How does he know when a bud is ready to harvest?

This is a question that's intrigued me. I've done my homework, and I even have some ideas on the subject. For instance, I'm thinking you could use mice.

That's not as crazy as it sounds. In the 1960s, there was a lot of interest in developing techniques to figure out how much THC and CBD were in marijuana buds. Recreational users were intensely interested, of course, because they wanted to know whether they were getting their money's worth. And law enforcement types were curious, too, because they wanted to know where the most potent stuff was coming from.

But that was back in the days before computerized chemical analysis. And it was long before the sorts of official marijuana testing laboratories like the one we'll visit in chapter 8. Instead, researchers developed all sorts of tests that would supposedly tell users what was in the buds they were buying, and which would let the cops analyze those buds when they confiscated them.

Of all of the tests that were used, I have two favorites. First, my runner-up is the peroxide-sulfuric acid test.[2] That test comes to us from research done in Yugoslavia more than half a century ago by Ljubiša Grlić. (The test he described was actually first suggested in 1938 as a possibility.) It goes like this: Take a piece of bud, then macerate it in petroleum ether (a mixture of petroleum by-products) for twenty-four hours. Then let that solvent evaporate and add a little hydrogen peroxide and concentrated sulfuric acid. (The result, alas, is no longer fit for human consumption.) Then . . . watch.

Through trial and error, Grlić was able to determine that this test produced different-colored liquids, depending on the bud's potency and mix of THC and CBD. For instance, he says, high-CBD buds turn pink, or even "blood red." THC, on the other hand, yields a violet color.

"As it is seen," Grlić concludes, "the peroxide-sulphuric test seems to be suitable as an indication of the progress of the ripening process in hemp resin." By the way, Grlić tested buds from all over the world. The most intense colors among the samples he tested came from Costa Rica.

Since I'm color-blind, I'll have to leave that test on the shelf. Fortunately, though, there's another test that doesn't require color vision. This makes it my favorite. That, plus the fact that this test's inventors promise that it's based on "the rather surprising taming effect of marihuana on aggressive mice."[3]

These researchers took mice one at a time and introduced an "intruder" mouse into its cage. The mice that attacked the intruder were selected as fighters. Next, the researchers injected those fighting mice with marijuana dissolved in alcohol, like the tincture used by Dr. John Clendinning, the sleep doctor of London. Then they watched what happened when intruders and the now-stoned fighters were reintroduced.

What happened—or rather what didn't happen—was their measure of a marijuana sample's potency, known as its ED50. In general, the ED50, or 50 percent effective dose, is the dose that's required to produce a 50 percent effect on an outcome. (In this case, fighting is the outcome.) So their ED50 was the dose required to produce a 50 percent reduction in fighting time.

Using that technique, the researchers were able to classify samples based on their ED50s. If we assume from what we've seen so far that it's THC rather than CBD that decreases fighting, these ED50 calculations would be a measure of THC concentration. A low ED50 would mean that a small sample was effective in calming those mice, so that sample probably has a high concentration of THC.

That's all well and good, but now I'm in Roger's dining room and I don't see any test tubes full of colorful liquids. Nor do I see any mice. And I certainly haven't seen any high-tech lab equipment. So he must have another way to figure out whether his plants are ready for harvest. But what?

"Well," Roger's voice booms behind me as he emerges from the narrow stairwell. "It's an art. But there's a little science to it. I'll show you."

Roger's dining room seems to serve as a study. Built-in wooden bookshelves line one long wall and are crammed with titles such as *Hemp and the Marijuana Conspiracy* and *Marijuana Reconsidered*. On the dining room table that serves as a desk is more clutter surrounding a compound microscope, like the kind they let kids play with in elementary school. There's an eyepiece lens and a choice of objective lenses that, at the lowest setting, give a magnification of about 30x. And that, Roger tells me, is all you need.

At first, I see nothing. Then I turn the focus knob, and long, thick tubes come partly into focus. They're too thick for the microscope to include all of them in the same depth of field. But by toggling the knob back and forth, what emerges is a cluster of what I'm guessing are trichomes.

"I just plucked these off this morning. What color are they?"

Well, they don't look like any color to this color-blind observer. Charitably, I guess you could say that they're whitish. But really, they're clear. This is what I tell Roger.

He says that if they're clear, they don't have much resin yet, so they don't have much THC. As they mature, though, they'll become opaque, turning white or amber or brown, depending on the strain.

And when does he think this crop will be ready?

"Not for at least a week. Maybe two." He looks wistfully at the microscope, as if he can't wait for those two weeks to pass.

You Know Ganja?

Although Roger tells me that a joint is his preferred method, joints aren't the best choice for everyone. Fortunately, there are lots of ways to administer the active ingredients of marijuana. One of the simplest would be to apply the stuff to whatever part of your anatomy is bothering you.

Wouldn't it be great if, instead of lighting a joint and inhaling, you could simply put marijuana's active ingredients on a sore knee, for instance? But is that possible?

That's a question I have an opportunity to answer on a long hike in Nepal, which was supposed to be unrelated to any marijuana research. This hike, to the hill station of Nagarkot, is not for the fainthearted. Or for the middle-aged. The trail starts at a bus station about ten miles from Kathmandu, and then it climbs. And climbs.

I've been on this trail for the better part of the morning, slogging along behind my fleet-footed guide Avinash. He's happily leaping from one stone step to another. I am plodding. Right foot. Left foot. Gasp. Repeat.

Although Avinash was initially amused by my distress, now it's becoming apparent that I'm slowing him down. At this rate, we're not going to get to the guesthouse until after dark. We've already had a spirited discussion about the merits of Nepali beer compared with foreign beer, and I know Avinash is looking forward to a Heineken or two that I've promised to buy him. Yet that frosty green bottle is a long way away.

I'm exhausted and sweaty, and the backs of my thighs are aching. But the worst discomfort comes from my left knee, which was injured in a playground accident many years ago. Every step sends a prolonged dull ache down into my foot and up to my hip.

Whenever we stop to rest, Avinash asks me a few medical questions that seem to be cribbed from a rudimentary medical textbook for Nepali guides.

"Where hurt?" "Can walk?" And, ominously, "Lie down?"

At about the fourth stop, Avinash seems to have gathered enough information to make a diagnosis.

"Old knees," he says with finality.

And his recommendation?

"How do you say . . . Poultice?" I nod. "Very strong medicine. It has . . . ganja? You know ganja?"

I certainly do. And I'm intrigued. Marijuana ointment? Really?

I've stumbled—literally—on a question that I've been wondering about for a while. I'm learning a lot about how marijuana works and what it does. But I don't know much about how to get it into people.

Today I have a chance to try Avinash's method, which, he promises, will make my knees feel better. But he says it won't make me high.

"No problem with head," he declares. "Keep on trail."

That's essential, because I really can't afford to get stoned. We still have eight miles to go, and I'm looking forward to that beer as much as Avinash is. So I'm intrigued by the idea that it might be possible to deliver the active ingredients in marijuana to a particular part of the body. Hopefully bypassing "head."

I nod.

Avinash flashes the happy grin of a dealer who has just made a sale. Which, I guess, is basically what he's just done.

About an hour later we reach signs of civilization. I hobble through a welcoming committee of dogs, and we're in the main street of a village that consists of perhaps a dozen houses on either side of a narrow dirt road. Then Avinash dodges through a gap between two cinder block huts and disappears through an open door. A second later, his head emerges and he beckons me in with a wave.

Now we're in a cool, dark room about 10 by 10 feet. It has a low ceiling, and its walls are lined with bottles and jars, interspersed with bunches of what look like dried herbs. Avinash gestures for me to sit on a bench just to the left of the door, and as my eyes adjust to the gloom, I can see we're not alone.

In the room with us is a woman of indeterminate age—somewhere between forty and eighty—who is pottering around a table against the far wall. She gives me a traditional *namaste* greeting that is de rigueur in rural Nepal. I return the gesture, and then Avinash and the woman engage in a rambling conversation in Nepali.

After perhaps two or three minutes of this, the woman turns back to her bench and Avinash turns to me.

"Says she has medicine."

The woman takes a battered tin off the shelf, pries off the lid, and hands it to Avinash, who hands it to me. I'm looking down at a dirty white paste with an overpowering smell of hydrocarbons, like kerosene.

"For knees," Avinash says. Then he points at the problematic parts of my anatomy, as if he doesn't quite trust his powers of translation. I'm pretty sure I'm supposed to rub this stuff on my knees.

This goop looks more like something you'd use to strip the grease off the clutch plate of a vintage Mustang than anything you'd smear on any part of yourself. But what have I got to lose? I take a modest finger's worth and apply it to my right patella. Avinash seizes the tin and smears generous dollops on both knees.

There's an initial sensation of intense cold and tingling. It feels a little like menthol-based ointments like Bengay. I'm guessing that is the kerosene or whatever is causing its awful smell. I'm probably highly flammable right now, and I resolve to stay away from open flames. That sensation passes quickly, though, and now I'm staring down at two greasy white knees that hurt as much as they did five minutes ago.

After a leisurely lunch of the ubiquitous *daal bhat* (rice and lentils), I try a nonchalant stroll to the pit toilet behind the house, only to find that this local remedy isn't doing much at all for my knees.

"We go?" Avinash asks.

We go. But in the first few hundred yards, I'm disappointed that the benefits of this stuff—if indeed there are any at all—are modest. We still have eight miles left to walk before we get to the guesthouse, and I have two tired knees.

This trial was disappointing. Especially for poor Avinash, who had to wait until well past dark for his beer. But it wasn't surprising.

Generally speaking, it's difficult for molecules to cross the skin. Our bodies are carefully constructed to keep our insides in and the outside world out. Indeed, there's a lot riding on our ability to keep these fortifications intact. So the skin is built in layers of cells with tight links between them. And the outer later—the epidermis—is designed as a physical barrier. It's made up of lots of cells that die quickly, so we're also protected by a thin, flexible wall of dead stuff.

We don't know a lot about how well cannabinoids are absorbed through the skin, but the simple answer is "not too well." For THC in particular, absorption seems to be low, unless you use high concentrations. Alternatively, you can dissolve cannabinoids in something like di-methylsulfoxide (DMSO) or another "permeation enhancer."[4] (DMSO is a powerful solvent that has a ninjalike ability to sneak across cell membranes, carrying other molecules along with it.) Indeed, there is a patent for a cannabinoid-containing patch that uses a gel containing permeation enhancers such as alcohols or glycerides.[5] It's a little like a nicotine patch, only significantly more fun.

Without a little extra help to get through the skin, though, THC and CBD are likely to stay outside. However, there is some evidence that CBD absorption might be considerably higher than that of THC.[6] That's interesting, because, as we've seen, some researchers are intrigued by the possibility of using CBD to treat pain.

In the future, there might be a new, better way to get drugs absorbed through skin. It's called an ethosome—basically a tiny lipid sac that contains a high concentration of ethanol. Think of it as a liqueur-filled truffle, about 100 to 200 nanometers across. (A nanometer is one billionth of a meter, so an ethosome that is 100 nanometers is one one-hundredth the size of the smallest human cell.) These ethosomes aren't quite small enough to get through pores in the skin, but the alcohol inside them helps to liquefy the skin's keratin layers, opening those pores just a little wider. And these ethosomes have shown potential as a way to deliver cannabinoids.[7]

However, without those high-tech truffles, the skin is a barrier that is almost impermeable. So if you want to get THC or CBD into people, you need another route. Just smearing it on the skin isn't going to do it.

Sativa Stout

Fortunately, there are other options. Lots of them.

What if it were possible to dissolve marijuana's active ingredients into beer? That wouldn't solve the problem of delivering it directly to the area on the body where you need it, such as a sore knee. However, THC and CBD dissolved in beer would obviate the need to light up.

And most of my patients—even those in the last days of life—can take sips of liquid. But is that possible?

After a little research into the matter, I learn that it is possible to make marijuana-laced beer. But there's a catch. When I ask people about the usefulness of this option, I'm surprised by their main concern. They're concerned about the taste.

Brewing beer involves a boiling step, and it's safer to add marijuana (or other ingredients) to a batch of beer before you boil it. Marijuana in particular often has all sorts of bacteria on it, which come by way of the dirt in which the plants have been grown, or from the hands of whoever picked them. By adding marijuana to beer before you boil it, you can kill those bacteria. However, when marijuana is added at that stage it imparts a muddy, dirty taste.

On the other hand, you could add marijuana after the boiling stage, and the taste will be better. But those bacteria won't get killed off by the boiling process, and they're going to grow and thrive. Until you drink them.

Marijuana-infused beverages prove to be rather difficult to find, but after some searching, I have finally located someone who has some experience with them. Even better, he has a couple of bottles of marijuana-infused wine and beer. His name is Jerry, and he's willing to share.

As we talk on the phone to arrange a meeting, I'm effusive in thanking him for sharing his liquid stash. But Jerry is surprisingly dismissive. "Don't thank me," he warns, "until you try this stuff."

This weekend Jerry's three daughters have gone to New York with his wife, and as we sit down on his back porch he seems to be reveling in the silence.

After some preliminaries, including strict promises not to reveal anything about him, Jerry disappears inside and reemerges carrying a dark brown 16-ounce bottle with a plain silver cap. It has a hand-printed label that says "Nirvana." The bottle also sports a sticker with alternating yellow and black rays—the international symbol for radioactivity.

Jerry opens the bottle and pours us each a sample into two small tumblers. The beer is a deep, dark brown, like Guinness. We clink glasses.

"The guy I got it from said he made it using a stout recipe. Lots of sugar. He was hoping that would mask the taste."

Did it?

"Don't get your hopes up."

I sniff first. It has a bouquet of compost. But old, dried compost that's burned out to become rich, smelly dirt.

I take a sip, noticing as I do that Jerry has put his glass down untouched.

It's sweet, I'll give it that. But the sweetness does absolutely nothing to mask the sour taste of grass and mud and wood shavings. The result is a little like drinking Kool-Aid out of a Wellington boot that's been used extensively for barnyard labor.

One sip is going to have to be enough. So, honestly, I can't report whether there was any psychoactive effect at all.

I look at Jerry, who shrugs. "Told you. At least that was the last bottle. Now I feel like I've done my duty."

Jerry dumps both of our glasses onto the ground underneath a hydrangea bush and rinses them under a spigot.

"But this should be interesting."

He picks up another bottle that's been sitting in a corner of the patio, up against the house. It's a regulation-size wine bottle with a plain white label that appears to have been computer printed. Not that there's much on it. There's the word *Special* in the flowing cursive beloved of winemakers. And the volume (750 milliliters). And the grape mixture: 40 percent Cabernet Franc and 60 percent Pinot Noir. And the alcohol content (13.5 percent). But that's it.

I note that the bottle is already open.

"I don't drink much wine," Jerry admits. "But my buddy said you should let it breathe." He pauses, considering. "Well, I figure it's breathed enough, don't you?"

I agree, and Jerry pours. Again we clink glasses. But this time Jerry doesn't put his down. That's a good sign.

I take a sip. Then another. It tastes, well, like wine. That's about it. Granted, I'm not the sort who waxes eloquent in flowing sentences about how a particular vintage is round and full-bodied, with layers of oak and hints of currant and blackberry. So my vocabulary is decidedly limited. Nevertheless, I'm pretty sure that if there were notes of cannabis, I'd detect them. I do not.

For the record, neither does Jerry. He pokes his nose into the juice glass about as far as it can go. He takes a deep sniff, thinks for a moment, then shrugs. Then drinks.

"Wine," he says.

That about sums it up. But, truth be told, we're not here for the taste. So we sip. And wait. And sip. And wait.

We talk about the news, and upcoming state elections as the level in the bottle gradually descends. After about an hour, we've each had two hefty glasses and the bottle is pretty much dead.

And the result? I stand to stretch and test my coordination. I feel about the same as if I had drunk two large glasses of wine in an hour. Which is to say that I'm certainly in no shape to drive back to my hotel.

However, I can't say that I feel anything else. I turn to Jerry for confirmation. This is a guy who surely knows a buzz when he feels one.

"Buzz? Nah. I got nothing. You?"

I confess that I, too, got nothing.

"Man, I can't figure out why people drink wine. Stuff tastes like grape juice that's gone moldy. I'll stick to smoking."

I confess I'm surprised by these underwhelming results. This bottle, Jerry was promised, contains two pounds of marijuana added to the fermentation barrel. That sounds like a lot.

Jerry stands and stretches. Then he goes inside the house, leaving me alone on the back porch with the remains of the bottle of Special.

As I sit quietly, awaiting developments, I try to do the math in my head. A wine barrel is about 50 gallons, I think. And that's about 200 liters, more or less. And two pounds are about a kilogram.

OK, so that's a kilo (1,000 grams) of marijuana in 200 liters, or about five grams per liter. If a bottle is 750 milliliters, that's roughly four grams we've ingested between us, or two grams each.

This, I also happen to know, is a decent amount of marijuana. A small joint runs around half a gram. So at two grams per person, we've each ingested the equivalent of four small joints, or two big ones.

I check my math again to make sure. That's about right.

But it can't be. Even half a gram, or one joint, would knock me out. And two grams? Forget it.

As I'm thinking this, I realize that I've been doing all of these calculations in my head. And some part of my brain is recognizing that if I'm doing this math correctly, then the empty bottle in front of me probably didn't contain much marijuana at all.

Jerry is similarly unimpressed. I know this because he's reappeared carrying a water pipe, a dime bag, and a lighter.

A Tragic Waste of 2,000 Joints

The next morning, nursing a mild hangover, I pause to reflect. Those adventures in fermentation were, on the whole, pretty disappointing. But they provide a fascinating insight into the science of how to get the active ingredients of marijuana into people.

Think about the wine we tasted. If that truly was a kilogram of marijuana, and assuming about half a gram per joint, I arrive at a number that is both intriguing and daunting: 2,000.

That's the number of medium-sized joints you could roll from the two pounds of marijuana that went into that wine barrel. Lay them end to end, and the resulting line of joints would stretch more than 300 feet, or the length of a football field.

So what went wrong? Why did our share of a football field's worth of marijuana fail to have an effect? There are three answers to that question, and together they tell us a lot about how to administer a dose of the active ingredients of marijuana. And how not to.

The first answer is about something known as bioavailability. Basically, this is a measure of how much of a drug we're getting. It's a number that's calculated for all of the pills that we get by prescription or over the counter, and it's expressed as a percentage. A higher percentage indicates that a drug is more likely to go from your gastrointestinal tract into your bloodstream.

Take THC, for instance. The bioavailability of THC that you swallow is between 10 and 20 percent. That is, of a hundred THC molecules that pass your tonsils, fewer than twenty will actually make it into your bloodstream.

So the measure I was using—of how many "joints" are in a bottle of wine—is overly optimistic. If Jerry and I really had smoked a couple of joints each, the cannabinoids in those joints would have been much more likely to get into our bloodstreams (30 to 50 percent). So Jerry and I only got about half as much as we would have if we were each handed four midsize joints.

OK, but that would still be two joints each, yet neither Jerry nor I came close to getting high. I'm pretty sure that smoking two joints would have put me into a coma. This brings us to the second answer, which hinges on the way that our bodies metabolize cannabinoids.

If you inhale marijuana smoke, whatever THC is absorbed into your bloodstream from your lungs will be carried up into your head. No detours. However, if you swallow THC, it has to take a much more roundabout path before it finally gets to your brain.

First, it needs to pass through the stomach and get absorbed in the small intestine. Next, it will be carried by the bloodstream through the mesenteric veins that collect blood from the intestines. Those veins then coalesce into the hepatic vein, which runs through the liver. This is a key step for THC and indeed for many drugs, since this is where the liver's so-called first-pass metabolism takes place.

In the liver, THC goes through two modifications. First, it's metabolized to 11-OH-THC, which is just a minor change. This new molecule just has an additional oxygen and hydrogen atom (OH). It's the equivalent of slapping a new coat of paint on an old house, making it look a little different, but still easily recognizable. Indeed, 11-OH-THC still has all of the psychoactive effects that THC does, and it's at least as potent.

But the next step is a more fundamental change. While the 11-OH-THC is moving through the liver, some of it is metabolized to another version of THC, which has the unprepossessing name 11-nor-9-carboxy-THC. This is a much more significant modification, analogous to giving that old house a new roof and aluminum siding and a sunporch.

Just as that house would be unrecognizable, your body's cannabinoid receptors don't bind to 11-nor-9-carboxy-THC the way they bind to THC, so it doesn't have any of the psychological effects that THC does. This means that as your blood leaves your liver en route to your heart, then your lungs, and finally your brain, it's been stripped of most of its THC. It's also lost a lot of its 11-OH-THC.

The net result is that when you drink THC in the form of beer or wine, your brain isn't seeing every molecule that is in that bottle. Many of those molecules will get changed into new molecules (11-nor-9-carboxy-THC) that don't act like THC. That is, they don't make you feel stoned, and they won't relieve your pain or nausea. In fact, they won't do anything at all.

But that can't be the whole story, can it? Even if the THC in the four joints in my share of that wine had been reduced to the THC that I would have gotten in a couple of puffs of a joint, I'm pretty sure I would have felt something. And Jerry, who I would assume is much more used to marijuana, would have at least noticed an effect.

This brings us to the third lesson in marijuana dosing, and that's a matter of time. The THC that you take by mouth (as opposed to inhaling smoke) has to pass through your intestine, into your bloodstream, and through your liver. And as it travels, and as it gets metabolized, the peak dose spreads out.

To see how that works, imagine two cars approaching a tollbooth. Their drivers choose different lines, each of which is several cars long. A few minutes later, one car emerges. But the other driver isn't so lucky. That toll taker is having a bad day, and is a little slower. And one of the drivers up front forgot his wallet. So the second car emerges several minutes after the first. On a larger scale, imagine a hundred cars all arriving at the same time. A few will get out in a couple of seconds, whereas others won't make it through for ten minutes.

Gastrointestinal absorption of cannabinoids like THC and CBD—and indeed most drugs—works the same way. A few molecules of THC might get absorbed and pass through your liver in fifteen minutes. Other molecules might take an hour. And remember that less than 20 percent get through at all.

So rather than the quick spike of THC you get if you smoke a joint, when you take a marijuana product by mouth you get a long, drawn-out curve that slopes gently up, and then back down, just as those one hundred cars approaching a line of tollbooths will get spread out. At any point in time, your blood levels of THC or CBD are going to be relatively low—much lower than the brief, intense spike of THC that you get after a few puffs on a joint.

The World's Best Pot Brownie Recipe

There's a fourth reason why Jerry and I didn't succeed in getting high. It's this fourth reason that's the most interesting to me, because it suggests a much better way to deliver the active ingredients of marijuana. And that, after all, was the goal of our failed experiment.

The theory of marijuana-infused wine and beer seems straightforward. Put marijuana into a vat of beer or a barrel of wine, and then wait. Eventually the THC and CBD will dissolve. A little like making tea. Right?

Well, no. In order to induce the THC or CBD molecules to leave the bud, you need to give them a liquid in which they're soluble. But they're poorly soluble in water. So if you dunk a bud in water, its THC and CBD are going to stay right where they are. (This explains why the marijuana tea I told you about at the beginning of this chapter didn't do anything for me, either.)

Nor did we get much of a buzz from the beer or wine that Jerry shared. In fact, I regret to report that the kilogram of premium weed that sat in that wine barrel for a year or so probably emerged with most of its THC and CBD intact. Then someone scooped it out and threw it away. Two pounds of premium marijuana became compost.

So how do you get these cannabinoids out of the buds *before* you toss them in the trash?

You know the answer, even though you might not realize it. It helps if you think of a bud of marijuana as a dirty pair of overalls. These overalls are stained with oil, and you want to get the oil out. What do you do?

Well, you could put them in a washing machine and fill it with water. Then you could let them soak for a while. You could do that, but you wouldn't.

Why not? Because oil isn't soluble in water. The oil isn't going to detach itself from the cloth to which it's clinging. In order to get that oil out, you need to add something that oil *does* like to bind to, like soap.

Similarly, if you want to coax THC or CBD out of a bud, you need to give them the equivalent of soapy water. To do that, you have two options.

First, you can use alcohol. Ethanol is the most common choice, because it's drinkable. Other forms of alcohol, such as isopropyl (rubbing alcohol), work, too. But since drinking isopropyl alcohol can cause severe nausea, blindness, and brain damage, it wouldn't be my beverage of choice.

It's true that both wine and beer contain alcohol, but you need high concentrations to induce those cannabinoids to leave their bud. Beer (about 4 percent) probably doesn't have enough, and even wine (about 12 percent) won't be able to coax much THC and CBD out of a bud. To do that, it helps to use alcohol that's 50 percent or higher.

The second option is fat, or lipids. These are molecules that have long carbon chains that bind to THC and CBD, pulling them out of a bud. There are lots of lipid molecules to choose from, but since we're talking about medications and things you might conceivably want to eat or drink, then the list is shorter. The main ones are olive oil, shortening, or butter. There are also variants such as Indian Bhang that uses ghee (clarified butter). Already, you can begin to see some intriguing culinary opportunities.

To get the THC and CBD into alcohol or butter, there are a couple of methods that are scientifically sound. Both of which, fortunately, are feasible in a typical kitchen.

First, you can make your own cannabinoid-infused alcohol. Start with a couple of buds. Then take a pure form of ethanol, like vodka or grain alcohol. Throw the buds in, and let them sit for a couple of weeks.

Some aficionados suggest stashing the mixture in a freezer. They point out that as the buds cool, the water in them freezes. And as that happens, the water expands, breaking open the hard cell walls of the plant material that holds the cannabinoids. In theory, at least, that results in a more potent brew. Then you simply strain through a sieve and enjoy what is often known as "green dragon."

The process of getting cannabinoids out of buds into fat is a little more complicated, but not much. And this method is important, because it's the way to get THC and CBD into most food items. First, you need to chop up a bud into small pieces in order to maximize the surface area that will be exposed to oil or butter. Some chefs suggest using a blender or a coffee grinder.

Then you need to heat those pieces in oil or clarified butter for long enough to let the cannabinoids in the bud seep out. Finally, let the mixture cool, then pour it through a fine sieve to strain out the pieces. What you're left with is oil or butter with high concentrations of cannabinoids, which you can use in any recipe. In fact, this technique is the basis for what an expert has promised me is the world's best (and simplest) pot brownie recipe. We'll meet its author in the next chapter, and his recipe is on page 261.

Alas, although this method of dissolving cannabinoids in oil or butter is pretty simple, it will only get you so far. As we've seen, whenever you try to use a marijuana product in a food or beverage, you'll lose more than 80 percent due to bioavailability and the first-pass effect (the liver's tax, so to speak). And that reduced dose will be spread out over several hours, making it difficult to anticipate and control. It can also be difficult to standardize the dose you're getting, since batches of brownies, or marijuana-infused vodka, are going to vary from batch to batch.

Granted, these methods do work. For instance, that pot brownie recipe will deliver THC and CBD in amounts that are large enough to have an effect. And those brownies will work much better than the ointment I tried in Nepal. Still, there's room for improvement. Fortunately, there's another approach to getting marijuana into people—another delivery system—and it's one that we've known about for a long time.

How to Get a Goat High

If you were a highly trained physician in the 1830s, and you happened to find yourself stationed in sleepy, steamy Calcutta, you might have discovered a shortage of tasks that could occupy your finely tuned mind. You would have cast around for diversions. In the end, to keep yourself from going bonkers in the heat and boredom, you would have found a hobby.

This was the story of Dr. William O'Shaughnessy, who graduated from the University of Edinburgh in 1829 and then journeyed to Calcutta in 1833 as an employee of the British East India Company to work as a physician at the Medical College and Hospital. Soon after arriving in Calcutta, he decided to study the use of marijuana for medical purposes. Specifically, he decided to investigate "its utility in the treatment of tetanus and other convulsive disorders."[8]

However, there was a problem. In studying the benefits of marijuana, O'Shaughnessy needed to figure out how to get its ingredients into his research subjects. That proved difficult for two reasons.

First, O'Shaughnessy performed his initial tests on dogs and goats, and he knew that it would be difficult to encourage them to smoke a joint. Second, even if he could get dogs and goats—and eventually people—to smoke marijuana, there was no easy way to determine what dose his subjects would be getting. How much was in a puff? And was a caprine puff equal to a canine puff?

With typical British resourcefulness, O'Shaughnessy turned to the laboratory and made a tincture, just as Dr. John Clendinning's "medical man" in London in the 1840s did to get a good night's sleep in chapter 2. A tincture is a highly concentrated, alcohol-based solution of cannabinoids, like the vodka infusion mentioned earlier, but much more intense. Think of all of the cannabinoids in a joint dissolved in a few drops of alcohol. That's a tincture.

O'Shaughnessy proudly shares his recipe: "The resinous extract is prepared by boiling the rich, adhesive tops of the dried gunjah, in spirit (sp. gr 835), until all the resin is dissolved. The tincture thus obtained is evaporated to dryness by distillation, or in a vessel placed over a pot of boiling water."

That is, O'Shaughnessy boiled the marijuana buds in a beaker of ethanol. In the foregoing, "sp. gr 835" refers to the specific gravity, or density, of the alcohol ("spirit") he used. Pure ethanol has a specific gravity of 0.79 and water's is 1.0. So O'Shaughnessy's alcohol, at 0.835, is almost pure ethanol. Then, once the THC- and CBD-heavy resin was dissolved in the alcohol, he had a concentrated liquid that he could administer to dogs, or goats, or people.

Armed with his tincture, O'Shaughnessy was ready to proceed to animal trials. First up, a dog of "middling size."

> In half an hour he became stupid and sleepy, dozing at intervals, starting up, wagging his tail as if extremely contented, he ate some food greedily, on being called to he staggered to and fro, and his face assumed a look of utter and helpless drunkenness. These symptoms lasted about two hours, and then gradually passed away; in six hours he was perfectly well and lively.

Subsequent experiments shared the joy of ganja with a small dog, who became "ridiculously drunk." Next, three goats, only one of whom exhibited any effect at all—a "change of countenance." (I can only imagine what that looks like in a goat.)

Delighted with these dramatic effects, and convinced of ganja's safety, O'Shaughnessy concluded that it was time to move on to humans. One of the first recipients was a man named Hakim Abdullah. He had been bitten by a rabid dog three weeks previously, and presented himself to O'Shaughnessy's clinic in extremis.

"His eye was restless, suspicious, and wild: his features anxious; his pulse 125; his skin bedewed with cold moisture." In short, he was believed to be in the early stages of rabies, which typically has an incubation period of two to three weeks. Rabies causes, among other symptoms, a paralysis of the muscles involved in swallowing, producing an intense thirst but an inability to drink.

The good doctor noted that after the third dose his patient became cheerful. Soon, O'Shaughnessy reports, "his pulse was nearly natural; the skin natural in every respect; his countenance was happy." The only odd note, O'Shaughnessy admits, was the patient's rapturous descriptions of the ladies of his *zenana* (a room or wing of a house designated for women). O'Shaughnessy was able to determine, through sources that are better left to the imagination, that the patient's home was not so endowed. Nevertheless, the poor man's relief proved to be sustained, and continued dosing was successful in keeping the patient comfortable for five days, until he faded into unconsciousness and died, presumably still thinking of his ladies.

As a method of administration, tinctures are useful clinically. You can give them to seriously ill patients who are having trouble eating or drinking. And also to goats, if the need arises, or if you need animal volunteers for a research study.

There are two additional advantages of a tincture. The first is that you can titrate the dose with almost perfect accuracy. In any given batch, every drop in that flask has the same dose of THC and CBD. You can give two drops to one patient, and four drops to another, with the certainty that the second patient is getting exactly twice the dose of the first.

There is another advantage of a tincture. But it's one that O'Shaughnessy probably didn't appreciate at the time. Or if he did, he omits it from his reports.

Earlier I mentioned the "first-pass effect," the metabolic "tax" or diminishment of potency that the liver takes on drugs like THC that come in through the gastrointestinal tract. The impressive thing about a tincture is that it bypasses this tax, due to an anomaly in the way that blood flows through the GI tract. At either end—at the mouth and the rectum—some veins bypass the liver and go right back to the heart, and then out to the body.

By putting a few drops in a patient's mouth and allowing it to be absorbed, you're bypassing the first-pass effect. You can be sure that most of the THC in those drops is getting out into the body. And, of course, the onset of action is quicker, because you're not waiting for the THC to make its way into the intestine, then through the liver and into the bloodstream.

Despite his successes, William O'Shaughnessy still faced one enormous problem, which became apparent in his account of his efforts to treat rheumatism. (This is what we describe now as rheumatic fever, a secondary effect on the heart and joints of infection with a particular type of streptococcus.) He describes his experiments with three patients for whom all other treatments had failed:

> But little relief had been derived from a fair trial of antiphlogisitic measures, and of Dover's powder with antimonials; in the last case, sarsaparilla at first, and subsequently the Hemidesmus Indicus with warm baths had been tried without advantage.

You should know that in the 1830s, if you tried sarsaparilla and antimonials to no avail, you were really up the creek. Antiphlogistics, which could be found in willow bark, were primitive anti-inflammatory agents. Antimonials contained antimony, and were used to induce vomiting. *Hemidesmus indicus* was a plant used in Ayurvedic medicine and doesn't seem to do much of anything. And sarsaparilla is good in soda with a twist of lemon.

When all of those treatments failed, O'Shaughnessy reached for his tincture. He gave exactly the same dose to all three patients. Two hours later, one became "very talkative, was singing songs, calling loudly for an extra supply of food, and declaring himself to be in perfect health."

But that's only part of the story. "The other two patients," O'Shaughnessy admits, "remained unaffected."

So what was the problem? Why did one patient get totally stoned when the other two were untouched?

The answer is bioavailability. That's the measure of how much of a drug gets into the bloodstream and—ultimately—into the brain. I told you earlier that the typical bioavailability for THC or CBD taken by mouth is between 10 to 20 percent. But those figures vary between people. A lot.

A group of researchers discovered this when they gave twelve subjects a tincture containing THC and CBD in alcohol (as in the drug Sativex).[9] They sprayed it into the subjects' mouths, just as O'Shaughnessy did for his rheumatic fever patients. Those researchers were surprised to find a ninefold variation in peak plasma concentrations of THC. That's a ninefold variation with the same dose, administered in the same way.

We don't know why there's such wide variation among people. Maybe anatomical differences in the way that blood vessels are distributed in the mouth cause faster or slower absorption. Or maybe those different blood levels are caused by factors the researchers didn't measure.

With such variability in effects with the use of tinctures, perhaps it's not surprising that Dr. O'Shaughnessy's advice to other physicians is rather modest. In a warning, he tells potential users, "the practitioner has only to feel his way, and increase the dose till he produces intoxication as the test of the remedy having taken effect."

Beer and Brownies?

Despite all of William O'Shaughnessy's efforts to make marijuana dosing scientific, in the end he admitted that caution was needed. We need to start with low doses, he suggests, and increase slowly. That's a long way from the sort of standardized medical practice that he was hoping for.

Worse news, perhaps, is that his caution applies to all of the methods we've met in this chapter. Whether you're using a tincture you bought at a marijuana dispensary, or brownies you made yourself, it's almost impossible to be sure of the "right" dose. And that's a problem because, as we've seen, absorption using these methods takes a while.

Especially when the cannabinoids are in food, they have a long way to go before they reach your brain. So that's a long time to wonder whether you gave yourself the right dose or whether, maybe, you should have another brownie.

That's a problem, but it's hardly a fatal flaw. Certainly there are other drugs such as morphine for which there is no predefined recommended dose. I've taken care of some patients for whom a modest 15-milligram pill twice a day was enough to keep them comfortable. But I've also taken care of patients who required more than 1,000 milligrams per day intravenously.

I didn't choose those doses by reading the morphine package insert, but rather through a process of trial and error, the same process that O'Shaughnessy describes of starting with a low dose and increasing carefully.

But that trial and error process works best if you know what you're getting. So, of all of the ways I've shown you of administering precise doses of THC and CBD, tinctures seem like the best bet. Sure, there's some variability in absorption. But there's probably less variability with tinctures than there is with brownies, or with other edibles that are susceptible to the first-pass effect. And unlike beer and wine (and lotion), at least you're getting some.

Absorption is also quicker, since the THC and CBD are absorbed directly from the mouth into the bloodstream. From there they reach the brain and other organs quickly—much more quickly than they would if they had to travel through the intestine and then through the liver.

Granted, that speed isn't essential for relief, and sometimes a drug's slow increase and plateau in blood levels can provide sustained benefits. But a quick peak does make it easier to predict when the maximum dose will hit. Within the first thirty minutes or so of using a tincture, you'll have a pretty good idea of whether your pain or nausea are better. And if they aren't, you can use some more.

The other advantage of a tincture is the one that motivated O'Shaughnessy's experiments: reliability. Each drop of a tincture contains the same amount of THC and CBD. So if one drop was effective in relieving your pain or nausea, you can be confident in using the same dose again. That's close to the kind of reliability that you can expect when you pick up a bottle of antibiotic pills at the pharmacy, and much better than eating a brownie—or two—and hoping for the best.

It probably makes sense to use marijuana as an edible, too, but only if whoever is making those brownies or chocolates or potato chips knows that you need to use lipids or alcohol to extract the cannabinoids from marijuana. And even then, absorption can be variable, and delayed. So it will probably take more time—and work—to get to the right dose of an edible. You'll also need to be careful about variation from day to day, since the cannabinoid concentration in brownies, for instance, is probably going to be a little different from one batch to the next.

Finally, there are other methods that probably don't work. Ointments, for instance. And beer and wine. Also tea. Sure, it's possible that you'd absorb some THC and CBD using these methods. But probably not enough to be effective.

5

Bongs and Budder

As we've seen, it's possible for people to get the active ingredients of marijuana by consuming beer and brownies. And that works. But it's hard to know how much you're getting, and it's hard to predict when that dose will kick in.

So it's worth learning about how we can inhale those active ingredients.

I'm not talking about the tried-and-true methods of smoking a joint or taking a hit from a bong. Sure, you could do that. But the science of inhaling cannabinoids is actually much more complicated, and much more interesting, than firing up a joint.

There are much more advanced methods, such as the vape pens that Rachel and Jason used. There are even industrial-sized vaporizers that, according to their marketing materials, are "great for parties!" There are also different forms of marijuana that can be inhaled. Hashish, for instance, is a sort of concentrated resin made from the parts of a cannabis plant with the highest levels of THC and CBD. And there are even more concentrated substances such as "budder" that can be smoked.

Steve and the Volcano

To find out whether some ways of inhaling marijuana's ingredients are more reliable than others, I've sought the expertise of someone who knows a lot about all of these tools of the trade. Steve has tried them all, and—even better—he's promised to show me the future of marijuana inhalation.

The first thing I notice when I walk into Steve's apartment is that the plain wooden table just inside his front door is stacked with incoming mail that's been carefully arranged by size. This neat little parade of envelopes sits between two large and elaborate glass bongs.

This combination of neurotic neatness and pervasive marijuana worship is the overarching theme of Steve's apartment and, I suspect, his life. The living room is spare and almost barren, but punctuated by the bright bursts of Technicolor marijuana posters that line the walls. There are bongs and vape pens everywhere. This could be the apartment of an obsessive-compulsive bong tester for *Consumer Reports.*

And that's a pretty good description of my host. Steve is thin and wiry, with sinewy forearms and a deep tan that looks like it's been acquired through years of outdoor labor. He's clean shaven, with a blond crew cut, neat polo shirt, and creased khaki shorts. Although he looks like the last person in the world who would be an expert on marijuana, a physician colleague told me that Steve is more knowledgeable about medical marijuana than any patient—or physician—she'd ever met. So Steve, it seems, is the perfect person to show me the future of medical marijuana.

That future arrived by mail yesterday, sent via FedEx to Steve's apartment. By the time I arrive, he's already unpacked what he refers to reverently as "the device." After he lets me in, he takes me out onto the apartment's small patio that offers a panoramic view of a parking lot and a gas station, as well as a distant glimpse of the Pacific. There's a small, rough wooden table, and on it is a plate of brownies.

I have to ask: Are those . . . ?

"Oh yeah. Want one?"

I'm thinking that a dose of THC-laced baked goods will not do much to enhance my scientific fact-finding. So I pass.

The reason I'm here is an aluminum cone about 10 inches tall and 10 inches wide at the base. It looks a little like a volcano. And that, it turns out, is its name. This device, Steve has assured me, is the future of medical marijuana.

And that future consists of vaporizing.

Vaporizing, Steve explains, is the best way to extract THC and other cannabinoids from marijuana. "It's pure," he says. "It's free of contaminants." And, in a flight of poetic license, "It's the true essence of what marijuana can be."

Coming from anyone else, this lyrical ode would sound just plain silly. But Steve is a careful guy. His copies of *High Times* are filed chronologically. He's not the kind of person to take a leap of faith regarding any new marijuana technology that comes along.

So vaporization is a cleaner way of smoking?

"No, it's not smoking at all," Steve says as we sit down, eye to eye with the Volcano between us. "Marijuana that's vaporized doesn't burn. That's the beauty of it."

"When you burn the weed, you inhale everything," he explains. "The THC, sure. But also the fiber and dust and other chemicals and tar." He pauses. "And, you know, legs."

Legs?

"You know, from insects."

He means that when you harvest a marijuana bud, you're harvesting whatever happens to be there. And when you smoke it, you're smoking whatever happens to be there. He makes a disgusted face, as if he's describing sucking on the dirty end of a vacuum cleaner.

"With vapor technology," he continues, "you basically turn the cannabinoids to vapor that you inhale. And you leave everything else behind, where it belongs." He looks at the Volcano with a bright gleam in his eyes. "It's amazing."

And it is. Vapor technology is based on the principle that cannabinoids like THC evaporate at a cooler temperature than what's required to burn the marijuana. So vaporizers heat the marijuana to 180 to 200 degrees Celsius (roughly 355 to 390 degrees Fahrenheit). That's hot enough to vaporize THC and CBD, but not hot enough to cause the marijuana to burn, which happens around 230°C (around 446°F). So the fiber, tar, and insect legs stay behind.

I carelessly suggest that vaporizing is a little like smoking crack. Crack cocaine vaporizes at about 80°C (about 175°F), far below the temperature at which any impurities would burn. So heating to that temperature provides a pure vapor and an immediate, intense high.

Steve looks at me as if I've just suggested he's a crackhead.

I try a different analogy. Maybe it's more like extracting alcohol from a still? Ethanol boils at about 78°C, and water boils at 100°C (212°F). So if you heat a still to 85°C, then you can collect the alcohol as vapor, leaving water and other stuff behind.

Steve nods. "Exactly. It's a purifying process."

It's also potentially more than that, though, he explains. THC vaporizes at 157°C, but CBD vaporizes at 180°C (about 355°F). THC, remember, is responsible for the psychoactive effects of marijuana. So by choosing a temperature that's higher than the vaporization point of THC but lower than that of CBD, you could enhance those effects. Conversely, you could dial in a more mellow high by boosting the temperature to vaporize more CBD, giving yourself a mix of THC and CBD. In theory.

But I'm still thinking about the purification process. What about, you know . . .

"Water pipes?" Steve has anticipated my question. I nod.

"No, it's a myth that water pipes give you a cleaner smoke."

How could that be? You "wash" the smoke and what emerges should be . . .

"Not much different than regular smoke, actually," Steve says. "Sure, you get rid of some particulates and some tar. But here's the thing: You also get rid of THC. I mean, like, a lot of THC. So you cut down tar by 10 percent, but you have to take twice as many puffs. So you're actually getting 80 percent more tar."

I confess I'm not keeping up with Steve's calculations, and I'm more than a little skeptical. This is a guy who smokes pretty much every day, so how sharp could his brain be? But later, armed with the calculator on my iPhone, it turns out that Steve's math is correct.

So if a strain of marijuana is 5 percent THC (a typical concentration), then a vaporizer will extract about 50 percent of that THC. Compare that to about 30 percent of smoke from a joint. A water pipe is probably between 10 and 20 percent.

That's what led Steve to the Volcano. He's tried other vaporizers, but the Volcano has apparently gained a reputation as being the best. Its website and associated how-to videos extol its virtues in providing a clean experience, without tars or particulates. But lest that seem too scientific, the website also lets loose, describing the Volcano as being able to fill a nine-foot-long balloon, making it "perfect for parties!"

Despite that little burst of exuberant marketing, the website and promotional materials generally walk a thin legal line. Overall, the Volcano's website reads as if it's been vetted by a roomful of attorneys. For instance, the company refers primly to the customer's "material" and describes the Volcano as an "aromatherapy device."

Aromatherapy? I guess that's technically true. But my hospice offers aromatherapy to our patients, and I'm pretty sure I've never seen one of these devices before. I hope my nurses stick with lavender.

Steve and I are joined by his friend Bruce, who has apparently read the official *Big Lebowski* handbook on How to Look Like a Chronic Marijuana User. He's heavyset, with an unkempt beard, frayed T-shirt, baggy cargo shorts, and flip-flops. He looks like he spends his life strolling from one high to the next. He's here, Steve told me, because he's always been a skeptic of the Volcano, but now he's ready to be convinced.

"Oooh, brownies!" Bruce says. He turns to me. "Steve makes awesome brownies."

Bruce opens a rucksack and pulls out a dime bag of marijuana, and then a small, battery-powered music player that he sets on the table in front of Steve. He presses a button and the sounds of Johnny Cash's album *I Walk the Line* fill the patio.

Now it's time. Steve plugs the Volcano into a wall socket and Bruce looks on with the sort of wide-eyed expectation of a baseball fan on opening day. Then Steve leans over and presses a red button. A yellow light comes on, indicating that the heating element is warming up.

Steve taps another button, to set the temperature to 200°C. (I learn later that the Volcano comes in both analog and digital models. It should come as no surprise that Steve happily paid $100 extra for the digital version, which he says offers "added precision.") All three of us watch the Volcano intently as its temperature climbs slowly but steadily toward the 200°C target.

Steve picks up a small, cylindrical object from the table. It looks like a small nutmeg grinder. Apparently you can't vaporize marijuana in its natural state. First, Bruce explains, you need to grind it.

"You can't use whole buds," Bruce says, "because they're too large. They have a low ratio of surface area to volume."

He's referring to a general principle of physics that the smaller any object is, the more surface area it has for a given volume. That's why finely ground coffee makes a stronger brew, for instance. And why powdered sugar dissolves faster than granulated sugar.

So the smaller a piece of marijuana is, the more surface area it has per gram. And that's important, because you need surface area to let the heat vaporize the cannabinoids. More surface area means more cannabinoids, and Bruce doesn't need to explain that more cannabinoids are a good thing.

Steve adds a small pinch of Bruce's marijuana to the grinder. It's about half a gram, he tells me, or about what you'd put in a modest joint. Then he grinds with a practiced twirling motion of one wrist.

That takes him no more than a few seconds. Then the Volcano's yellow control light blinks off, indicating that it's ready for action. Steve and Bruce simultaneously break into grins.

The Volcano has a filling chamber, which is basically an orange plastic ring that sits over a wire mesh base. It looks a little like the trap that sits in the drain of a sink. Steve fills that chamber about one-third of the way to the top and tamps it down gently.

"You don't want to get it too tightly packed," he explains. "But you want to get it even. You want all the particles mixed up and about the same size."

Steve sets the chamber on the peak of the Volcano. Then he snaps on what he says is the control valve, topped by a thin, flat plastic bag. Right now, this little vaporizing device looks like a cartoon robot head with a plastic Mohawk.

Bruce and Steve look at each other and nod. It's a solemn moment that brings to mind two officers simultaneously verifying nuclear launch codes. Then Steve presses the green button.

Launch is a go.

The superheated air is blown through the little canister of weed and vaporizes any cannabinoids in that carefully ground sample. A second later, the little wedge of plastic begins to unfold into a balloon about 10 inches wide and 24 inches long. It's sticking straight up.

The balloon fills quickly, and Steve presses the green button again to stop the fan. He removes the balloon and I'm surprised that what's inside doesn't seem smoky at all. There's just a light fog. He turns it upright, with the valve pointed at the ceiling, and proffers it to me. I decline.

Next, he offers it to Bruce, who hesitates, then shakes his head. This is your baby, his gesture seems to say. The honor, my friend, should be yours.

So Steve takes a small puff, smacking his lips as you might if you were tasting a particularly complex '78 Château Lafite Rothschild. Then he takes another small sip, nodding.

Then Steve takes a drag that seems to empty half of the balloon. Despite claims about the pulmonary damage incurred by long-term marijuana habits, clearly Steve's lung capacity is still in great shape.

Holding his breath, he hands the balloon to Bruce, who skips the tasting preamble and inhales the remainder of the bag's contents. I am impressed. Between the two of them, they seem to have the combined lung capacity of a horse. Then Steve exhales slowly, and Bruce follows suit.

"Smooth," Steve says.

"Very," Bruce agrees.

They ponder those nuances for what seems like a full minute. I'm starting to feel left out.

"Are you getting it?" Bruce asks no one in particular.

"Oh yeah."

Vapor Science

This tasting has obviously been a success. But Steve and Bruce's enthusiasm for vaporizing may not be entirely warranted by the science behind it. At least, what little science there is.

It turns out that vaporizing doesn't extract more THC than, say, smoking a joint would. We know this because Donald Abrams, the San Francisco oncologist I spoke with about using cannabinoids to treat cancer, conducted a study that compared vaporizers with joints. He gave twenty-one active marijuana users the chance to get high, but in exchange they had to give blood and urine samples.[1] That seems like a fair trade, but they also had to agree to be hospitalized for six days during the trial. Apparently that was a problem for at least one subject, who was summarily ejected because he was unable to adhere to the research center's "rules of comportment."

Abrams found that people who used a vaporizer didn't have any more THC in their blood than did those who smoked a joint. Any differences weren't significant, and the curves of THC doses were essentially the same. So a vaporizer probably won't get more THC into your bloodstream than a joint will. Also, the total dose, measured in blood levels over time, is pretty much the same for a vaporizer and a joint.

However, that study did find lower levels of carbon monoxide in the air that subjects exhaled after using a vaporizer, compared to smoking a joint. Granted, Steve and Bruce are not particularly worried about their carbon monoxide intake, but it's not something you want to get too much of. (Even in low doses, it can cause headaches and nausea and dizziness.) So, score one for vaporizers. And, as Steve pointed out, vaporizers should also eliminate users' exposure to other contaminants, such as insect legs.

There was a third result that doesn't have much to do with vaporizers, but which is fascinating nonetheless. Abrams tested three strengths of marijuana, with varying concentrations of THC (1.7 percent, 3.4 percent, and 6.8 percent). You'd think that the more potent marijuana would produce higher blood levels of THC, whether people were smoking a joint or puffing on a vaporizer. But you'd be wrong.

In fact, the curves of THC blood levels over time look pretty similar at each of those concentrations. And, as THC concentrations increased, each milligram of THC in a joint—or in a vaporizer—is actually less likely to end up in your bloodstream.

How can that be?

One answer is that people using marijuana may modulate their intake from minute to minute based on how they feel. That was a common theme for many of the patients I interviewed for this book. Particularly Rachel, the woman who used a vape pen a couple of dozen times every day, titrating its effects to manage her pain. Indeed, Abrams found that when his subjects were given higher concentrations in a vaporizer, there was a trend toward less intensive "puffing behavior."

Incidentally, people who roll their own joints also titrate their dose. A British study of 247 users found that they were pretty good at adjusting the size of the joints they rolled, according to their marijuana's THC content.[2] Users with high-octane marijuana tended to roll smaller joints, and vice versa. Because CBD doesn't have psychoactive effects, users didn't seem to be aware of their marijuana's CBD content and didn't factor that in when deciding to roll a fat or skinny joint.

How the subjects in Abrams's study modulated their dosing is more of a puzzle. You'd think that perhaps they inhaled less deeply, or held their breaths for a shorter period. But in this study, subjects were held to the "Foltin uniform puff procedure." Subjects took five seconds to inhale, ten seconds to hold their breath, and forty-five seconds to exhale before repeating. So any modulation was due to rather subtle changes in breathing, and perhaps the number of puffs.

There's another feature of the science of vaporization that would have interested the long-departed Dr. O'Shaughnessy in Calcutta. We saw that he observed considerable variation in his subjects. One man started singing, but another was unaffected.

It turns out that whatever benefits the vaporizer might offer to acolytes like Steve and Bruce, it won't do much to reduce that variability. Abrams's vaporizer study I just mentioned found even greater variability in peak concentrations among these subjects.[3] One person experienced a peak concentration of a whopping 813 nanograms per milliliter. Granted, that was with the marijuana that had the highest THC concentration (6.8 percent). But even using that high-test weed, another poor soul only managed to achieve a peak concentration of 22.5 nanograms per milliliter.

Another measure of THC concentrations, the "area under the curve," is calculated to adjust for the fact that some people might absorb THC at different rates. It reflects the dose that people get over a period of time, so one person might get her peak THC concentration after two minutes, while another might take ten minutes, but they'd have the same area under the curve. Still, though, in Abrams's study this measure varied more than tenfold.

To put that in perspective, consider a study that was done on the drug fentanyl, an opioid like morphine. Researchers used an aerosol delivery system that let patients inhale fentanyl, where it was absorbed in the lungs and passed into the bloodstream, just as THC and CBD are. That study found a roughly threefold variation in both peak concentrations and the area under the curve.[4] Abrams's vaporizer study, remember, found a tenfold variation.

So this is a problem. In fact, it may be one of the biggest problems that the medical marijuana movement is going to face. Not knowing—by a factor of ten, how much of a drug you're going to get makes it almost impossible to find the right dose for the right patient. And it's really difficult to do rigorous research when you don't know for sure what dose your subjects are getting.

Vape Anywhere!

There may be a solution to this problem, and it's one that Steve knows a lot about. But he's staring glassy-eyed at a wedge of the Pacific that's visible in the distance. So I'm going to have to wait a bit. Bruce is still having trouble formulating complete sentences and is staring at a red pickup truck parked in the lot beneath us.

Finally, Steve surfaces enough to pronounce the effects of the Volcano as "mellow" but "intense." Then he's back among the living, and he tells me about vaporizer pens. Or "vape pens," like the one that Rachel used to manage her pain, and which Jason (the young man in chapter 3 who looked fabulous on chemo) used to control his nausea.

The theory behind the vape pen is exactly the same as that of the Volcano, he says, with the convenience of small size and portability. They're pen-sized devices in which batteries power a heating element that vaporizes marijuana-infused oil. Steve pads inside and comes back out with one that's about five inches long and an inch thick, made of black plastic. He opens a compartment to show me where the ingredients go.

I admit it looks portable. And indeed, their advertisements promise that they "fit easily in a briefcase or purse."

"Vape anywhere!" they suggest.

OK, I understand the attraction of vaping anywhere. But because the main problem we've seen with smoking and vaporizing and tinctures has been variability in dosing, I'm wondering how vape pens can solve that problem.

The answer is counterintuitive. It's possible that vape pens may provide better dosing because they don't work well. Each puff doesn't deliver nearly as much THC or CBD as a puff on the Volcano does. You need lots of tiny puffs to get the same effect.

And that's good, because lots of tiny puffs mean that a user can titrate the dose. It's similar to the difference between a drug like morphine that can be administered in a pill or in an intravenous infusion.

In pill form, you absorb a lot or a little, so you either get an adequate effect or you don't. You just take the pill and hope for the best. But with an infusion, it's possible to check back every few minutes and increase (or decrease) the dose as needed. These pens provide little bursts, and users can take one puff or thirty. All together, or spaced out over time.

We don't know much, yet, about what these vape pens actually deliver. Most of what we know comes from studies of e-cigarettes. The technology and theory are pretty similar. In an e-cigarette, you're basically using a small battery-powered heater to vaporize a chemical (nicotine) that's been suspended in a mix of oil and propylene glycol.

Do e-cigarettes work? Well, if by "work" you mean they deliver nicotine to the bloodstream, then it depends. Some studies have found that they do, in doses that are roughly equivalent to a cigarette.[5] But other studies have found that at least some models don't deliver much at all.[6]

If you translate those results to the newer fad of vape pens, one lesson is that the buyer needs to beware. Not all pens are equal. However, a more positive message is that if at least some e-cigarettes are effective, then maybe vape pens can be, too.

Cherry Tomatoes Versus Hamburgers

I ask Steve and Bruce if they're fans of vape pens. Steve shakes his head, and explains that the doses are too variable, and he has trouble getting a good buzz. But Bruce says he likes them.

"I like the control, you know? That's super important, considering my density."

His density?

"I've got a lot of extra pounds. So all that adipose tissue sucks up the THC. Lets it out slowly. So I need to control the dose up front."

What he means is that he has a bigger-than-average reservoir for THC. Remember that cannabinoids like THC and CBD are soluble in fat. All of us have fat in our bodies—some more than others. The more adipose tissue you have, the more THC and CBD you'll store.

In fact, because of these fat reservoirs, THC can be detectable for at least a week after the last dose.[7] THC concentrations may even go up after people stop using, due to its release from fat. Granted, Bruce doesn't need to worry, because those levels are still quite low. It's not as though he's going to take a couple of puffs on a joint on a Saturday night, and then suddenly start feeling a buzz on Wednesday morning.

This delayed-release phenomenon works in the brain, too. In an autopsy study, researchers compared levels of THC and metabolites in the blood and brains of twelve recently deceased people. They found that even when THC was undetectable in the blood, it was present in significant amounts in the brain.[8]

The good news is that you do have some control over when your stores of THC are released. At least, if you believe one ingenious experiment in which researchers took rats and fed them THC.[9] Lots of THC. That produced happy rats.

Then they stopped giving the rats THC, presumably making them less happy. As they did, the rats' blood levels of THC, and its metabolite THC-COOH, declined. Finally, the researchers stopped feeding the rats entirely.

When those rats stopped eating, they did what most creatures do— they started breaking down fat. And as that happened, blood levels of THC-COOH started to go back up. (A side note of that study was the finding that an injection of adrenal corticotrophic hormone, a so-called stress hormone that also promotes fat breakdown, had the same effect.)

In a similar study in people, fourteen regular marijuana users were put on a stationary bike for thirty-five minutes and their cannabinoid levels were monitored.[10] That brief burst of exercise caused an increase in both cannabinoid levels and free fatty acids (a breakdown product of fat). Moreover, that increase was proportional to subjects' body mass index—a measure of obesity. Bruce's THC levels presumably would have gone up quite a bit.

To be fair, one other study in people found that neither fasting nor exercise would increase THC levels enough to affect drug test results.[11] And all of these studies were done over a couple of days. So a former pot smoker who goes on a crash diet a year after his last puff is not going to get stoned.

Still, it's pretty clear that adipose tissue is a storage depot, and that people with more adipose tissue store up greater reserves. So hours after a puff, they may still have detectable blood levels. That's actually helpful if you want to try to even out a dose over time. But if you want control, or especially if you want to make sure you're clearheaded by tomorrow morning, a reservoir isn't such a good thing.

That's why Bruce is a fan of the vape pens, he explains. He thinks they let him administer just as much as he wants, when he wants it. It's better, he says, than a big dose all at once that's going to get stored in adipose tissue.

"It's like eating cherry tomatoes."

It is?

"Sure. You eat cherry tomatoes all day, with just a few calories each, and your body burns those calories gradually. But if you have a cheeseburger, that's more than you can metabolize at once, so all of those calories go to your gut."

I don't have the heart to point out that, given his admitted "density," the tomato strategy has not been particularly successful for him. At least in theory, though, Bruce might be right. THC and its metabolites would be pushed into adipose tissue by a difference in concentration. Higher blood concentrations would tend to push more THC into fat.

However, I can report with confidence that Steve is not interested in the vape pen, which has been unceremoniously tossed back into the living room where it's landed—amazingly—on the couch about 15 feet away.

Now Steve is reaching for the grinder. He's ready to set up another batch. He asks if he should add some for me.

I decline.

But Steve seems forlorn, and on my way out the door, he hands me a small paper bag containing a brownie sealed in plastic wrap.

Umm, is this going to get me in trouble going through airport security?

"Nope. No problem. It's just a brownie."

"Steve makes really great brownies," Bruce reminds me.

"I'll even give you the recipe." (He did—it's on page 261.)

In the long security line at the airport, I have ample opportunity to contemplate the wisdom of running the gauntlet with Steve's brownie. But then I have a vivid image the reaction of the US Airways flight attendants if, somewhere over Kansas, like O'Shaughnessy's patient #1, I begin "singing songs" and "calling loudly for an extra supply of food."

I decide to pass, and as I toss Steve's brownie in the trash, I'm comforted, at least, by the knowledge that my two hundred fellow passengers won't be treated to my rendition of Johnny Cash's "Hey Porter" over and over, for the next five hours. I hope they're grateful.

The Hash Artisan

As we've seen, there's wide variability in dosing when you smoke or vaporize or eat a pot brownie. And the dose you get is spread out over minutes or hours. That makes it difficult to get the right dose, and almost impossible to get a large dose quickly.

What if there were a way to get large dose of THC or CBD, quickly and reliably? Drugs like morphine can be given intravenously in a hospital or hospice to achieve this, and cannabinoids can be given intravenously in a research setting. For the average medical marijuana patient, though, that's not possible.

But there might be an answer. It's called hash. And I'm about to learn how to make it.

Hashish is a highly concentrated extract of the cannabinoids in marijuana. It can be smoked or mixed into food, or even rolled up into a little ball and swallowed like a pill. And because there's so much THC and CBD in a small amount, it's easier to establish a predictable dose.

My guide for today's lesson in making hash is Justin, a whip-thin African American in his early forties who is wearing a bulky wool sweater, cargo pants, and long dreadlocks. I was referred to him by a friend who works for a hospice in this city. She told me that Justin provides high-quality hash to some of her patients, and that he makes only small batches, without artificial chemicals. In short, he's a maker of artisanal hash.

We're in the kitchen of his apartment on the first floor of an old Victorian house in a sketchy neighborhood. The yard next door has an Oldsmobile on blocks in the front yard, and the house across the street has a new Cadillac in the driveway. It's a neighborhood that's either waiting for its rebirth or on its way down.

Justin's kitchen is a wide-open space that seems aggressively utilitarian. It's more like the food prep area you'd find in a nursing home than a kitchen where you'd make pancakes on a Sunday morning. There's a large aluminum mixing tank in a corner and boxes and plastic jugs lining the shelves. A massive steel-topped prep table sits in the middle of the room, with two fifty-gallon drums tucked underneath.

As he shows me around, Justin tells me he'd always been a recreational user of marijuana. But when he developed spinal stenosis several years ago, he started using more heavily to relieve the pain in his lower back and the spasms in his legs. From there, it was a natural move to begin growing and selling, and making hash. He tells me this matter-of-factly, as if anyone with back pain would, at some point, start breaking bad.

Justin explains that hash is made from the parts of the plant that are richest in cannabinoids. Specifically, it's made from lots and lots of trichomes. Whereas a bud in its natural state might have 5 percent THC, the trichomes that are stripped off might have more than 50 percent. (That figure proves difficult to fact-check, but chemical studies of trichomes do indeed show that they're packed with THC and CBD.)[12]

These trichomes are most dense on the buds. But as Roger the marijuana farmer explained, they appear elsewhere, too. Even on leaves and stems. No one wants to smoke those parts, but if you can somehow strip off those trichomes, you can use them to make hash.

As Justin is explaining this, I suggest that using the trimmings for making hash is a little like using leftover pork products to make scrapple. Justin's scowl suggests that this analogy isn't resonating with him.

"No—that's all just by-products. Junk. I mean, what's in scrapple? Who knows? Hash is like the opposite of scrapple." He pauses, as if he's thinking about the implications of that statement, and perhaps its appropriateness for a bumper sticker. "I mean it's pure. Nothing artificial. Nothing added. No chemicals of any kind."

I'm beginning to realize that purity is the creed he lives by. For instance, butane is commonly used to extract cannabinoids from trichomes, especially in large-scale operations. But Justin isn't having any of that.

"You'd use lighter fluid to make something you're going to eat? Or smoke? No way, man. Never gonna happen."

Justin uses ice water separation, and that theory is simple. Cold makes the trichomes brittle, so a little stirring breaks them off.

"Then you've got to separate the trichomes out." He pauses. "But that's easy, because—"

Because they float?

Justin looks at me as though I've said something appallingly stupid. "No, they sink."

He shakes his head. "Look, I'll take you through the process."

He turns back to an oversized white plastic cutting board on the counter and a pile of marijuana leaves. There's a large metal mixing bowl that's heaped with another bunch. I point out that there aren't any buds.

"No, not in this batch. This is just leaves. Skuff."

Justin scoops up a fistful of leaves. They've been dried, which means the inactive acidic THCA and CBDA have been converted to active THC and CBD. He dumps them into a fire-red institutional Vitamix blender and pulses it for a few seconds. Then he shakes the leaves into another mixing bowl. They're about the consistency that you'd use for basil destined to garnish a bowl of fettuccine.

A few minutes later, Justin pours about five pounds of crushed ice into a five-gallon bucket. Then he pours the chopped leaves into the bucket.

Now he's going to mix?

Justin shakes his head. "No—you're going to mix."

He fits a metal contraption onto the top of the bucket. It's got a large handle on a crank that protrudes to one side. I mix.

It's easy, relatively pleasant work. There's not a lot of effort involved, and indeed whenever I'm overly enthusiastic Justin reminds me to be gentle. I mix for about fifteen minutes, and when he lets me stop, I look down to find that the water is a dirty brown. Justin nods approvingly.

He places a mesh bag into a second bucket, explaining that it has openings about 200 microns wide. Together, we pour the mixture into the second bucket, and then he pulls out the mesh bag and squeezes. What's left in the bag looks like soggy tea leaves.

That's hash?

"No, that's junk." He tosses the bag in the sink to be cleaned and reused.

What we're looking for is in the bucket, he says. It had been brown water a moment ago, but it's starting to settle. Now there's a yellow-brown layer forming at the bottom.

Next, Justin reverses the process, pouring the brown water back into the original bucket that's been rinsed out. This time it's lined with a much smaller filter, which has openings of about 73 microns. It takes us at least ten minutes to squeeze the water out. But finally, the sediment is inside the bag. He turns the bag inside out, and scrapes the fine residue off with a flat piece of plastic.

This produces a pile of golden-brown mud in a mound about three inches wide and a half inch tall in the center. It has, he assures me, a THC content of about 50 percent. (The typical yield of this process is hash that is less than 5 percent of the original weight. A little higher if you use leaves, or lower if you throw in stems.)

Is there a way to increase the purity to 80 percent? Or higher?

Justin smiles. "Oh, you mean budder. Sure, I can do that."

Budder, Shatter, and Wax

Justin's promise of super-high-grade hash is of medical interest for two reasons. The first is reliability. Increased potency means increased reliability.

Think about it this way. If you have a drug that's 50 percent pure, that leaves a lot of leeway. Maybe one batch is 50 percent, but another might be 60 percent or even 70 percent. That may not seem like much, but imagine that variation as a proportion. Seventy percent instead of 50 percent is a *relative* increase of 20/50, or 40 percent.

To put that in context, imagine that you're taking a blood pressure medication at a dose of 100 milligrams per day. Then imagine that some days your pill contains 140 milligrams, and other days you get only 60. The FDA, of course, would never approve that drug. Hopefully you would never take it.

There is also the issue of purity. If hash is only 50 percent THC, then what's the other 50 percent? A pill might have fillers like starch or sugar. But what's the filler in hash? It's resin, and plant material, and gunk. Not exactly reassuring, is it?

So there's a medical reason to try to concentrate cannabinoids like THC and CBD as much as possible. But how?

The answer, it turns out, is a series of products that are like hash, only much more concentrated. And like hash, they're made in similar ways.

Just as Justin and I made our batch of hash by freezing the trichomes off plants, now he's about to show me how to freeze more quickly and more completely. The result, he promises, is going to be THC-heavy resin that is almost entirely devoid of other substances.

To do this, an ice-water bath won't work. One alternative is liquid butane. But as Justin pointed out, that's the stuff in cigarette lighters. Not only do you not want to put that in your body, but many inexperienced would-be hash artisans have been seriously burned or even killed when they've messed around with butane. It's not Justin's method of choice.

Instead, he uses liquid carbon dioxide. CO_2 in its normal state—at room temperature and normal pressure—is a gas. But if you chill it enough, it becomes a solid that we know as dry ice. It can only be a liquid under specific conditions.

Justin explains that if you can create those conditions, then you allow the liquid CO_2 to saturate the marijuana and drip through it. That's so-called supercritical CO_2, which exists in an ephemeral in-between state. As soon as the temperature warms up and the pressure drops, that liquid turns back into a gas, leaving highly concentrated hash behind.

Interestingly, the same technique is used to decaffeinate coffee. Earlier I mentioned that Donald Abrams and Barth Wilsey used "placebo" joints in their clinical trials: they were made using this process, or something similar. If you extract the THC and CBD from a joint, you're left with what is, literally, a weed.

What the liquid CO_2 extracts is rich in cannabinoids. Sometimes that's a fine powder that looks like what you'd get from an ice-water extraction. Or a wax that is called "wax." Or the hash oil that Cal and Cindy gave to their daughter Randi, that's called "oil." Other names, like "budder" or "shatter," are not as obvious but reflect the product's consistency, which can range from a gooey mud to a glasslike substance that looks like peanut brittle.

But what do you do with it? I'm about to find out.

Justin has already admitted that all of this work is making his back pain worse, and he was contemplating smoking a joint. But my interest in budder prompts him to offer a demonstration of what it does.

Now we're in Justin's dining room, a strangely Zen space with only a few original watercolors on the walls and a bare plank farmhouse table in the center.

Justin takes a small two-ounce glass jar out of a cupboard. Then he takes out his "oil rig," which looks like a modified Erlenmeyer flask that has an arm sticking out at a 45-degree angle. That arm ends in a small glass cup that holds a plug and a tiny titanium screen. He pours spring water (of course) from a ten-gallon jug in the corner into the flask. Then he places a small chunk of budder on the screen.

Justin disappears into the kitchen and reemerges with a blowtorch that looks exactly like what you'd use to caramelize sugar. Although I'm pretty sure we're not making crème brûlée.

We've already discussed my participation in this activity, and I've decided emphatically against. But I'm curious to see what sort of effect it's going to have on Justin.

At first I figure it might not have much of an effect at all. The piece of budder on the screen is about the size of a raindrop, with a volume of about a milliliter. And that's roughly a milligram. Even at 100 percent THC, that seems like a tiny dose.

But even a milligram of THC could have a huge effect, because it's going straight to Justin's brain from his lungs. There's no first-pass effect at all. Any THC in that little piece of budder is going to arrive in Justin's brain within a second or two of his first toke, and all at once.

Now Justin is showing me how this is done.

"You've got the dab of budder on the screen, right?"

Right.

Justin picks up the blowtorch. He fires it up and a narrow blue flame shoots out two inches. He trains it on the piece of budder, which begins to bubble. Then it starts to smoke. Justin kisses the opening at the top of the flask and takes a short breath. Then a longer one, drawing the smoke magically down into the flask, where it bubbles up and disappears into his lungs.

In less than ten seconds—the blowtorch off and safely sitting on the table—Justin is staring glassy-eyed at a point about twelve inches above my left shoulder.

Thirty seconds later, he's still staring.

This mental intermission gives me a good opportunity to think about the use of Justin's rig as a delivery mechanism for medical marijuana. However, I really don't need that much time to decide that this is a nonstarter for most of my patients.

Why?

First, there's the blowtorch. I just can't see myself writing a prescription for anything that requires an open flame.

And—let's be honest—this is just a little too close to smoking crack.

I can see its appeal for recreational purposes. But for most patients who are looking for relief of symptoms like pain or nausea, it seems like it's likely to be a turnoff.

But my biggest concern is sitting right in front of me. Justin looks like someone has taken a hammer to his skull. It's been a minute and counting. And he hasn't blinked. I ask him how he's feeling, and he doesn't answer me. One minute stretches into two.

Finally, Justin begins to return to the living.

"That's intense," he volunteers. He smiles and lapses into silence.

This is the problem with a form of marijuana that's almost 100 percent pure. Sure, the effect is reliable. But the peak is enormous, at least if you inhale it. There's no doubt in my mind that Justin is feeling OK right now, and that any spasms in his legs are long gone. Or, if they're not, that at least he's not caring a lot about them.

But this seems like overkill. It's a little like using general anesthesia for a headache.

To be fair, there might be situations in which a concentrated dose would be appropriate. For instance, some of my patients have severe pain associated with wound dressing changes. Others have discomfort with procedures like a bone marrow biopsy. I could imagine using something like budder for those procedures. There would be an intense high that wouldn't last long. And, for a short period at least, you wouldn't need to be functional. So I'm not discounting budder entirely.

Still, for general medical use, I'm not seeing it.

I thank Justin. He smiles. I ask him if I can get in touch with him later if I have questions. He keeps smiling. I decide I'll let myself out.

Bongs and Budder

If Justin's oil rig is overkill for most situations, then what's the best way of inhaling, for those people who want a quicker, more reliable dose than they can get from edibles or tinctures? There's smoking, for instance. And vaporizing. And vape pens. And hash and budder and oil.

The verdict? Some form of vapor delivery seems like the most reliable. Especially vape pens. I know their effectiveness varies, but they deliver THC so quickly that users have complete control over the dose they get and when they get it. Current models aren't particularly reliable, and they take some coordination to use. But those sorts of usability problems seem eminently solvable. I'm optimistic that we'll see more and better vape pens in the not-too-distant future.

Tabletop vaporizers like the Volcano are pretty neat, too. Their promise of delivering cannabinoids without inhaling smoke is a big plus. If you can get THC and CBD into people without inhaling smoke, that's a good thing.

Finally, I wouldn't dismiss budder and its highly concentrated cousins. Although it is difficult to see how they could find a role in general medical use, there are situations where a very brief, extremely intense dose could be useful, possibly including painful procedures like wound dressing changes. Or maybe it could be used for other medical or surgical interventions that cause some discomfort and a lot of anxiety, such as dental procedures.

I'll admit that makes budder a solution without a clearly defined problem. And maybe it won't be a good fit for any of the difficulties my patients encounter. But as with so much of the science of medical marijuana, I think it's worth keeping an open mind.

On the other hand, there's a note of caution here, too. I'm still thinking about Justin, sitting in his dining room and staring vacantly at the ceiling. That relatively small dose of THC incapacitated him entirely, taking his brain off-line. Sure, purity is great, if it helps patients know how much THC or CBD they're getting. But watching that effect should make us wonder about what kind of damage marijuana might be wreaking on our brains.

6

Reefer Madness

It's starting to look to me like marijuana might offer real medical benefits. For pain, certainly. And nausea. And probably other symptoms, too.
So I'm becoming convinced that marijuana is really "medical."

I confess that's a surprise. When I started this journey, I really didn't
think that marijuana had much medical benefit at all. But I've been
impressed by the stories I've heard from patients, by the studies I've
read, and by the researchers I've spoken with.

But impressed enough to use marijuana myself to treat a medical
problem? Well, that's a different question. Even if there are medical
benefits I didn't expect, there are still risks.

Throughout my medical training, I've been hammered by warnings
about marijuana and other drugs. It causes schizophrenia, I was told, and
depression. And it's addictive. And it's a "gateway drug" whose use will
lead inexorably to the abuse of stronger and more dangerous street drugs.

Nevertheless, I've been impressed enough by marijuana's medical
benefits to give it a try, for medical purposes. I'll tell you about that experience. The results are impressive, interesting, and more than a little
scary.

That experience turns out to be the perfect introduction to the next question we need to ask about medical marijuana: Is it safe? Or is it as safe, at least, as other drugs that are available?

In this chapter, I'll take you on a tour of what we know about the psychological risks of marijuana. I'll tell you what we know about the risks of mental illness, for instance, and of addiction. I'll also introduce you to the dangers of driving under the influence.

The Perils of Dancing Patio Furniture

I've just been kicked in the back by a horse. An enormous, muscular horse with an anger management problem.

What's worse, this isn't just an angry horse, it's a vindictive one. If I move just a little bit, I get the breath knocked out of me. If I twist just a tiny bit in the wrong way, or breathe, or cough . . . wham!

If you've reached a certain age and if you've experienced the misery of a lower back injury, this description should sound familiar. If you haven't, then now you know what you have to look forward to.

For me, an ill-advised attempt to lift a canoe precipitated my first encounter with this psychopathic horse years ago. But that first encounter wasn't the last. I've reinjured my back several times over the years, usually for something silly and trivial. This encounter with the horse was precipitated while shoehorning myself into a tiny midlife crisis convertible, which I'm now planning to list on eBay for a quick sale.

As I mentally say good-bye to my car, the horse gives me another kick, and again the pain is instantaneous. The initial stab of pain is followed—as I knew it would be—by a twisting agony that seems to draw the muscles in my back tighter and tighter like the wringing out of a wet towel. I can feel my back growing iron hard in the space of a minute.

Six months ago, I would have reached for a bottle of oxycodone. And, if it weren't 7:00 a.m., a large glass of bourbon.

Now, though, I'm thinking seriously about marijuana as a potential remedy. And why not? I've reviewed the evidence, and talked with enough researchers and patients to suspect that marijuana might relieve pain.

It's time for some minor-league self-experimentation.

Alas, medical marijuana is not legal where I live. This makes official testing difficult. Fortunately, however, I have friends. And those friends have friends. And one of those friends arrives at my door an hour later bearing the sort of resealable paper bag that's used to store a pound of French roast. And indeed this one probably did, not too long ago. I poke my nose inside, inhaling the aroma of coffee beans, and discover two joints.

"Happy to help," he says cheerfully. "Hope you feel better. I have to run—have to get to court."

That gives me a moment's pause. I hadn't stopped to consider the legalities of the experiment I was about to try. Had he been arrested?

He smiles. "No, I'm a lawyer. I do trusts and estates." He names one of the most prominent white-shoe law firms in the city. He pauses. "But be careful. That stuff is strong."

Well, I hope so. In the past two hours I've taken 1,200 milligrams of ibuprofen and two leftover oxycodones, with no effect whatsoever. So much for modern medicine.

I collapse into an Adirondack chair on the back porch. It's still early on an August morning, so it's not too hot. I hold up a moistened finger. There's a nice breeze blowing from right to left. That's convenient, since the house to my right is occupied by a Baptist minister. The house to my left is occupied by a couple of doctors who I hope have already left for work.

Cradled by the chair, I strike a match.

I take one puff. Then another. Nothing. Then I inhale a few more times in rapid succession, using the "Foltin uniform puff procedure," which, as mentioned in the previous chapter, consists of five seconds to inhale, ten seconds to hold a breath, and forty-five seconds to exhale.

A moment later, I feel a vague sensation of light-headedness. Like vertigo, but much more enjoyable. It's like the patio furniture and shrubs and trees around me have all taken a couple of steps back. They're leaving. Going on a vacation. I smile for the first time in the past two hours. Good for them.

However, these introductory puffs have done absolutely nothing to dull the pain that's still twisting the muscles in my back. And even the most minor shift in position—there—causes a spasm that's so torturous I almost drop the joint that I've been holding far too casually.

Desperate for some relief, I take another toke, but am interrupted by a fit of coughing that induces my back muscles to go into a spasm all over again. When that passes, finally, I realize that the joint has burned about halfway down. After a few more hits, there's still about a third of the joint left, but I decide it's wise to heed my courier's warning. I pinch it out with moistened thumb and forefinger and set it aside.

And I wait.

As I do, I notice that my back seems to be loosening, just a little. My muscles are conforming reluctantly to the chair's curve. Maybe that's the oxycodone kicking in. Or maybe it's just my imagination. But I really do feel a little more relaxed. I'm thinking the travails of middle age might actually be manageable.

This is the moment when things start looking up. This is also the moment when things start to get weird.

My first clue that my world is going sideways is the behavior of the tree off to my left. It's a great big, gnarly yew that gives my backyard a distinguished Middle Earth feel, as if any moment a hobbit might appear on one of its branches, singing a homesick ode to the Shire.

But not now. Now it looks like it's guarding something. Actually, it's guarding *me*. It's looming over the deck, ready to drop one of those heavy branches on my head if I make a careless move.

I'm also distracted by the voices that are coming from inside the house. Where there shouldn't be any voices. Because there aren't any people. And yet there are, unmistakably, voices floating out through the open windows behind me.

What's slightly more disturbing is the topic of their conversation. These unexpected guests seem to be talking about . . . planes. Specifically, they seem to be air traffic controllers. And they're directing planes in the air, from my living room.

Is the Federal Aviation Administration aware of this? I'm guessing not.

Then there are the deck chairs in front of me, which seem to be made of silver. I decide I like the look. Sort of like what you'd get if Walt Disney redecorated the Playboy mansion.

Their little feet are skittering over the cedar planks under them in time to a rhythm that only they can hear. Or maybe I could hear it, too, if only those air traffic controllers would shut the hell up.

It's at this point that I fall asleep. Actually, it's a weird, waking dream in which I float in and out of a fleeting awareness of my surroundings. It's like part of my brain decides to put up a periscope every once in a while and check on things.

That lasts for a long time. I'm not wearing a watch, but when I check a clock inside much later I figure I was out for about three hours.

My return to the real world is gradual. The first clue to my reentry is that I realize I'm hot and thirsty. The sun had been hidden behind the malevolent yew, which is now just a tree seriously in need of pruning, but is now full on my face.

I move reflexively—and too quickly—to swat a mosquito, and the spasms in my back return with a new ferocity. I wince, but it passes more quickly than I expect.

Interesting. Make a note of that.

I listen intently, and I am unaccountably sad to realize that the air traffic controllers seem to have vacated the premises. Such a pity. I'll miss them.

After my head has cleared, I take stock of my interesting morning. The sterling-silver deck chairs were nice, I guess. And it was comforting to know that all of my air traffic control needs could be met by simply hollering in through my living room window. But I would have preferred to get some relief without those side effects.

Shrinking Brains

If you've ever witnessed the short-term effects of marijuana that I experienced, you have to wonder: What happens if those effects don't go away? What if a marijuana user continues to experiences those auditory and visual hallucinations, tinged with paranoia in the form of a looming yew tree? (If you haven't noticed those short-term effects, then you haven't been paying attention.)

And that lack of attention might be the most prominent long-term effect of marijuana use. There is at least some evidence that chronic marijuana users may lose some ability to retain new information—that is, to learn.[1] However, these deficits don't seem to be enormous. In fact, they might not even be large enough to be noticeable, outside of formal neuropsychological tests.

More concerning are studies that have found that marijuana could cause structural changes in the brain. In one large review of forty-three studies, researchers found an overall trend toward shrinkage in several parts of the brain. Those included parts of the cortex (the medial temporal and frontal areas), as well as in the cerebellum.[2]

Even more interesting—and concerning—are the studies in that analysis that used imaging tools like a functional magnetic resonance imaging (fMRI) scanner. An fMRI shows which parts of the brain are more or less active. Some of those studies found that the brains of marijuana users responded to thinking tasks differently than did the brains of nonusers.

That's worrisome. Just the possibility that marijuana is causing atrophy of some areas of the brain is pretty scary. And if marijuana causes changes in the way that brains work, why would anyone take that risk?

Well, to put that risk in perspective, some of the studies included in that review involved people who used marijuana for decades. And many used it heavily. Keep in mind, too, that all of these studies involved people who used marijuana recreationally. Some studies accounted for other drug use, but most didn't. So were those brain rearrangements the result of marijuana use? Or were they caused by other drugs, like cocaine or heroin or alcohol?

Another question is whether those changes matter. Granted, that's not a question you want to be asking. When we're talking about the brain, I would like to be sure that my own gray matter is working as intended. But what really matters is how those structural changes affect the way that a person thinks.

For one answer to that question, consider this study that put ten chronic marijuana users and ten matched controls through a battery of psychological tests. Then all twenty subjects were put through an fMRI scanner.[3] The researchers found that as the marijuana users were trying to remember recent information, one area of the brain—the left superior parietal cortex—wasn't working normally. But the researchers also measured memory and the ability to pay attention selectively, and they didn't find any differences. So those changes in the brain didn't seem to affect how those people were thinking, presumably because our neural pathways have enough built-in redundancies and excess bandwidth that modest structural changes don't impair thinking.

Even more intriguing is a study of fifteen long-term heavy marijuana users, and sixteen controls, that found that the users had a smaller hippocampus and a smaller amygdala compared to the controls.[4] The hippocampus and amygdala are areas of the brain that have a role in learning. That study also found that marijuana users did worse on verbal learning. However, there was no association between learning and brain volumes in either group, so people with more shrinkage didn't necessarily have more trouble learning. That is, there were changes in learning, and changes in brain volume, but those changes seemed to be unrelated.

Other studies have also found brain changes in young recreational users.[5] However, it's interesting that in this population, at least, gender matters. For instance, one study found that heavy marijuana use was associated with an increase in size of the brain's amygdala, but only in women.[6] Also interesting is one study's discovery that brain changes are more prominent in people whose hair samples contain a high ratio of THC to CBD, raising the possibility that CBD might protect against brain damage.[7]

It's important to keep in mind, though, that all of these imaging studies are pretty small, and a small sample makes it harder to find statistically significant relationships between marijuana use and brain function. So it's possible that there are real effects of marijuana use that would have been apparent if these studies had enrolled two hundred people instead of just twenty. As more research is done, with larger samples, it's possible—even probable—that we'll begin to see effects of marijuana on thinking, or on brain development and structure, or on both.

Of those two, it's the structural changes that are most concerning, even if they may not have any direct relevance to how we think. That's because the brain isn't good at repairing itself. Brains that are damaged tend to stay damaged. And a damaged brain is a serious problem, because a damaged brain may have less reserve capacity.

Think about the brain as a call center, full of workers answering phones. Now imagine that the call center downsizes to cut costs, laying off 30 percent of the operators. It can still function adequately, and callers don't notice a difference.

Now imagine that it's winter, and flu season hits. One day a third of the remaining operators don't show up. When there was a full complement of operators, that wouldn't have been a problem. But now, with a reduced workforce that was barely adequate, calls are going unanswered.

That's why we should be concerned about structural brain changes. Maybe those changes don't result in a decrease in function now. Maybe they're not even noticeable except in an MRI scanner. But as our brains age and lose some of their capacity, then structural damage becomes much more of a problem.

Putting all of this together, it seems likely that there are some long-term effects of marijuana use on the brain. At least some studies have found effects on thinking and memory. And then there are these changes in brain structure and function. It's difficult indeed to tell how those effects—if they truly exist—might translate to medical marijuana users. But in theory, at least, some effects on memory and attention seem plausible.

Reefer Madness

It's also possible that chronic exposure to THC might predispose people to mental illness. At least, that's what I was taught in medical school. In lecture after lecture, my fellow students and I were subjected to a grim litany of warnings about marijuana's psychiatric risks. And it turns out that there may be at least two genuine psychiatric risks.

First, marijuana might increase the risk of a psychotic episode. Patients who experience a psychotic episode often have symptoms that are similar to acute marijuana effects, but are not so amusing as imagining you hear air traffic controllers in your living room. Symptoms include hallucinations, delusions (often paranoid), or deranged and disorganized thoughts. There are enough reports of these episodes that we should take this risk seriously.[8]

If that doesn't make you nervous, here are two studies that might. Researchers in France followed 705 young adults between the ages of eighteen and twenty-seven for up to five years, tracking marijuana use and the incidence of psychotic episodes.[9] They found that increasing marijuana use over time was associated with increased psychotic episodes, and vice versa. Even worse, another study of 410 people who had experienced a psychotic episode found that marijuana users had that episode at a younger age.[10] The association was particularly strong for those who used high-potency marijuana.

That's not a causal relationship, of course. Maybe people with psychotic symptoms were self-medicating with marijuana. That could make it look as though marijuana was causing psychotic symptoms even if it wasn't. Based on the conversations I've had with patients like Tomas (the man in chapter 2 who suffered panic attacks after being kidnapped in Mexico), I think this is pretty likely. Also, in one study of 170 people at high risk of developing a psychotic episode, marijuana use didn't appear to increase that risk further.[11] Still, these results are worrisome.

The second reason to be concerned about marijuana use and psychiatric illness is probably the most important. That's the possibility that marijuana might increase the risk of developing schizophrenia, which shares many of the symptoms of a psychotic episode. However, whereas psychotic episodes are typically transient, and possibly a reaction to outside stress, schizophrenia is a chronic mental illness that can be personally, socially, and financially devastating. At least one good review has found that marijuana users might be more likely to develop schizophrenia, and particularly young men, who are already at increased risk.[12]

However, just as in the studies of psychosis, we need to be careful about drawing premature conclusions. Sometimes associations look concerning but turn out to be due to other factors. For example, in a study of more than thirty thousand people in Sweden, researchers found a strong association between marijuana use and schizophrenia.[13] That makes marijuana look dangerous indeed.

But once the researchers adjusted for family history and other drug use, that association disappeared. So there may be other causes of schizophrenia that might explain (and erase) what at first appears to be a clear case of cause and effect. In addition, other studies have found that marijuana use doesn't increase the risk of schizophrenia as much as a family history[14] or a history of childhood abuse do.[15]

Finally, marijuana may also have psychiatric risks that we just haven't discovered yet. For instance, it's possible that marijuana releases inhibitions enough to put people at increased risk of committing suicide. We don't know yet whether this is true, and in fact one study in Colorado didn't find an increased risk.[16] The problem, though, is that those researchers had to rely on county records of who registered to use marijuana medically, which probably substantially underestimated actual numbers. So their results are reassuring, but hardly conclusive.

At least the risk of psychosis, and possibly schizophrenia, are real enough to take seriously. That's probably especially true for younger patients who might use marijuana for years. I'm thinking in particular of patients like Tomas, who finally found relief for his PTSD symptoms with marijuana. I can't say that those risks outweigh medical marijuana's benefits for him. Maybe, for him, marijuana was still the best choice. But I'd feel better if I knew that he was aware of these risks, and that his family was, too, so they could be alert to new symptoms that might be signs of psychosis.

The Dangers of Marijuana and Guns

Although these psychiatric risks are uncertain, there is one risk that seems relatively obvious. Like many mind-altering substances, it seems likely that marijuana is addictive. But how addictive is it?

In order to answer that question, I'm looking at a pretty picture of a brain, in cross section. This particular brain belongs to someone who is addicted to marijuana, and most of it is a dull gray, displayed in hundreds of gradations. The detail is so fine that you can see the soft curls and edges of the brain's natural convolutions just under the skull.

I'm here to see these pictures of a marijuana user's brain, because this kind of imaging can teach us a lot about marijuana addiction.

I'm sitting in this pleasantly cluttered office at the Treatment Research Center at the University of Pennsylvania's Perelman School of Medicine in Philadelphia with Teri Franklin and Marina Goldman. They're both addiction researchers interested in studying brains like the one they're showing me. Franklin is a psychologist with wavy blond hair whose hair band and flowered dress give her a friendly earth mother vibe. Goldman is an addiction physician with dark-brown hair drawn back tightly from a face that's framed by almost invisible wire rim glasses. She's wearing a matching sweater set and slacks despite humidity and a temperature in the eighties.

They riff off each other constantly, finishing each other's sentences like longtime partners as they give me a crash course, in stereo, on marijuana addiction.

My education begins with my sheepish admission that I've never really thought about marijuana as being addictive. Not like cigarettes or cocaine, or even alcohol. And, if we're being totally honest, I've always thought about marijuana as being addictive in a humorous, *Harold & Kumar Go to White Castle* sort of way. More a burning desire to get stoned than a real life-destroying addiction.

Franklin and Goldman seem to have heard this skepticism before, and they have their talking points ready. Indeed, there's little doubt in their minds about marijuana's addictive potential.

"It's probably less addictive than other drugs," Goldman admits. "Only 9 percent of people who try it become dependent, compared with 12 percent for cocaine, and 15 percent for alcohol."

The word *dependent* is used to describe someone who uses marijuana regularly, even though it impairs their ability to function normally, and despite drug-related physical and psychological problems. People who are dependent may also experience withdrawal symptoms when they stop. (More about this in a moment; we'll return to Franklin and Goldman's tour of addicted brains below.)

That 9 percent sounds much higher than what I would have guessed. That's one in eleven people. But it might even be an underestimate. One study reports the prevalence of dependence in heavy users as being 21.7 percent.[17] A larger, nationally representative sample in the United States came up with an even higher number. That study found that 38 percent of users met criteria for dependence.[18]

If the risk of marijuana addiction is a surprise to you, it certainly was to me. But it shouldn't have been. We've known about the addictive potential of marijuana for a long time.

One of the first reports of marijuana addiction comes from an early description of marijuana withdrawal. (In the science of addiction, withdrawal symptoms are a hallmark of addiction.) That report dates from the 1940s when a British army physician named J. D. Fraser found himself responsible for the care of a regiment of native Indian troops who had been relocated.

While in India, those men had ready access to marijuana, but when they were mobilized for duty their supply was cut. We don't know what they had been smoking, but the withdrawal symptoms that Fraser describes were impressive. He summarizes common features in a way that would probably lead sober people to remain that way.[19]

"Irritability increased and culminated in a sudden outburst of violence, such as stabbing another man, striking out, or shooting at someone."

Shooting? Yes, these were soldiers, and they did have guns. Which, in retrospect, probably occurred to a few people as being rather ill-advised if they were also being allowed to smoke marijuana.

Fraser continues: "A common history was that the man had been on guard duty and had suddenly begun to blaze away with his rifle or Sten gun at an imaginary enemy. This sort of conduct," Fraser adds, "resulted in the man being brought under medical observation."

The other behaviors he describes are enough to give pause to anyone thinking of using marijuana or, I suppose, stopping. His patients "stripped themselves of all clothing and masturbated almost continuously; their habits became filthy, feces and urine being passed in the bed or on the floor."

Fraser describes other symptoms, including visual and auditory hallucinations, wandering attention, bizarre behavior, and fighting with other patients. "Some," he adds, "would sing at the top of their voices for hours."

Yet none died, a result that Fraser admits was surprising. And all were sent back to India where, presumably, they would resume their habit. "Clearly," Fraser concludes, "it would be safer if known cannabis indica addicts were not employed on foreign service."

Fraser was seeing a form of marijuana withdrawal, which I was surprised to learn is a real syndrome, recognized in psychiatry's diagnostic reference source, the *Diagnostic and Statistical Manual of Mental Disorders*, Fifth Edition (DSM-V).[20] Symptoms of withdrawal include anger or aggression, nervousness or anxiety, insomnia, decreased appetite, restlessness, depressed mood, and a variety of physical symptoms including stomach pain, tremors, sweating, or headache.[21] Studies have found that these symptoms are at their worst in the first four days, although people continue to experience withdrawal symptoms for more than two weeks.[22]

Going berserk and masturbating are not mentioned, but perhaps those behaviors would be subsumed under anxiety. Interestingly, the hallucinations that Fraser described aren't on DSM-V's list. In short, the good news is that this list is much more benign than what Dr. Fraser was so concerned about.

The bad news, though, is that withdrawal symptoms probably affect many regular marijuana users. One study of 384 attempts at quitting marijuana found that 40.9 percent of them met DSM-V criteria.[23] Of course, those were people who had been using marijuana recreationally, and were using enough for them to decide that they needed to quit. So occasional medical marijuana users would presumably have a much easier time stopping. Still, there doesn't seem to be much doubt that marijuana withdrawal symptoms are real.

Marijuana and the Addiction Circuit

But does the existence of withdrawal symptoms mean that marijuana is addictive? Addictive in the same way that cocaine, for instance, is addictive?

Back at the Treatment Research Center, Franklin starts clicking away on her MacBook, and the dull gray brains we were looking at a few minutes ago disappear. They're replaced with brains that are glowing. Each brain harbors bright splotches of yellow deep in their centers. These are fMRI images that create a visual image of what happens to the brain when a person is exposed to cues that can trigger craving for a drug.

Cues? Such as?

Franklin flips to another series of pictures. These images feature people who are smoking marijuana, laughing, and, in one vivid close-up, rolling a joint that looks to be approximately the size of a Genoa salami.

The technique they used in this study is actually pretty common in addiction research, they tell me. It's a way of looking for the circuit (Franklin's word) for addiction. These are the neural connections that are activated in response to a stimulus that makes someone think about using a drug.

"If you show these specific cues to someone who is addicted to a drug like marijuana," Goldman explains, "this is the circuit that lights up."

Franklin adds that the brain response is tailored to a person's drug of choice, and it often aligns with a drug craving. In other words, a marijuana-addicted brain will light up in response to an image of a large joint, but not necessarily an image of an ice-cold martini.

OK, I get that. But all I'm looking at is a little glowing dot inside a little gray brain. Where is this circuit?

Everything that motivates behavior ends up in the mesolimbic system, they explain. The mesolimbic area is in the center of the brain and extends out to the prefrontal cortex. This is the part of the brain that responds to pleasurable rewards, like getting high or tipsy. And so it's this part of the brain that prompts us to fire up a joint, or open a beer.

Goldman adds that this circuit can be activated in response to a cue, even if the person is unaware. Someone may feel "funny" but not understand that what they're experiencing is craving for a drug. And yet that person's brain is lighting up as if all it wants to do is light up.

Addiction researchers are hoping to develop imaging tools as a diagnostic test for addiction in order to find biological evidence that addiction exists. Goldman and Franklin see this circuit light up in other drug addictions, such as alcohol, heroin, and cigarettes. There's even interest in this circuit for behavioral addictions such as eating disorders.

If the same circuit lights up the same way in response to images of addictive substances like alcohol, cigarettes, cocaine, or heroin, and that circuit also lights up in response to images of marijuana, what does that tell us about marijuana and addiction?

"It's the same addictive process. It's the same biological marker across different addictions," Goldman says. "In the brain, these various addictions look pretty much the same."

How it works is complicated, but the short version is that this addiction circuit is created by a rapid rise and fall of the neurotransmitter dopamine in the mesolimbic area. When you sip a martini or take a drag on a cigarette, the mesolimbic area of the brain rewards you by releasing a flood of dopamine, which makes you feel good. Then as you finish that martini or grind out that cigarette, your dopamine levels go back down.

"What determines the strength of an addictive substance," Franklin explains, "is the speed of the change in dopamine levels." The more rapid that increase, she says, and the steeper the subsequent decline, the more addictive a substance is. The more addictive a substance, the greater the chance that the system can be hijacked and used for the purpose of maintaining the addiction. Thus, the faster you'll develop this thing that I'm beginning to think of as the "addiction circuit."

Granted, the significance or intensity of that circuit in someone's daily life may vary widely. For one person who is using heroin, it might lead to an all-consuming craving. For someone else, the same circuit may produce little more than a nagging desire for another hit.

However, the outcome is disturbingly similar, whether you're using hash or heroin. The circuit is hijacked by the drug, which sets into motion the same processes of craving, drug seeking, and withdrawal. In short, addiction.

Addiction and Medical Marijuana

I'm still skeptical. I understand that marijuana is addictive, but Goldman and Franklin are talking about recreational users of marijuana. I'm interested in people like Alice or Rachel or Tomas who are using marijuana for medical reasons.

That's an essential distinction. Medical marijuana users have a different motivation, for instance. And they use in different settings, often with at least some medical guidance. Perhaps most important, for medical users, getting high isn't a social event. They're not doing it for fun. So maybe medical users have a lower risk of addiction?

Consider drugs like opioids that are used both recreationally and for pain management. There's a big difference between people who use opioids for those two reasons. For someone who takes a drug like oxycodone to get high, the risk of addiction can be substantial. But the same drug, used in appropriate doses for someone who has pain, is unlikely to be addictive.

And all the patients I've met seem to be doing well. Rachel and her neck pain, Tomas and his PTSD, Jason and his nausea. They're stable, at least. And marijuana seems to be helping them. Is there really a 9 percent or greater chance that each of them will become addicted?

Franklin and Goldman believe that there is, because they see addiction in biological terms. A big risk factor for addiction, they're saying, is the combination of a drug and a person's genetic makeup that determine your brain response. This is what Goldman describes as a "drug-host interaction." That is, if you get the right (or wrong) pairing of a particular drug with a person's genetic makeup, you've set the stage for addiction.

That's just the beginning, though. As I get them talking about medical marijuana, they begin thinking about other concerns, and come up with three in particular.

First, the concentration of THC in marijuana is increasing steadily. That worries Franklin.

"Back in the seventies, the concentrations of THC in pot were much lower. One or 2 percent. Now you can get joints that are 7 percent, or 10, or even higher. More THC means more dopamine ups and downs."

Goldman cautions that we don't actually know that, and Franklin nods. But they're agreeing that as concentrations go up, the risk of addiction is likely to go up, too.

Marijuana's THC concentration makes me think of another concern. I mention methods of smoking hash oil that provide really high doses of THC, in a rapid bolus. Pipes, for instance. And vape pens.

That piques Goldman's interest. "You mean, like e-cigarettes."

She seems stunned. And worried. With good reason, it turns out.

Goldman reminds me that any drug that causes a rapid increase in dopamine, and a subsequent rapid decrease, is particularly likely to lead

to addiction. The more rapid those changes, the more addiction specialists get worried. So with the creation of new forms of marijuana that
lead to rapid spikes, the potential for addiction becomes much, much
greater. That's particularly concerning for concentrates that are smoked,
such as shatter and dab. Especially when they're smoked, as Justin's
was, in something that looks like a crack pipe.

It's too soon to know for sure whether we need to worry about Goldman's concerns about concentrated oils. But in one study of 357 users,
people didn't report an increased incidence of accidents or overdoses.[24]
They did, however, report that over time they needed to use more to get
the same effect. That is, they believed that they were developing tolerance. Since people who develop a tolerance often increase their dose,
that's not good news.

There's a second reason why Franklin and Goldman are so concerned about legalizing medical marijuana. It's not as obvious as the
first. But it may be more important.

Goldman points out that when we legalize marijuana for medical
purposes, we're putting it into more hands than ever before. Sure, not
all of those people are going to become addicted. But some will—that's
certain. So even if the risk is only a conservative 9 percent, if you double
or triple the number of users, it seems plausible that the number of people with an addiction is going to increase proportionally.

Franklin admits that that's not a real risk for people near the end of
life, and she and Goldman seem mollified by that thought. But I'm not.
And they both seem genuinely surprised when I tell them about some
of the people I've met, such as Tomas, Alice, and Rachel. They are not
terminally ill, and many are in their twenties. So they have a long, long
time to use marijuana and to develop an addiction. And there's plenty
of time for that addiction to wreck their lives. I think I've just made
these two researchers very, very worried.

Then it's their turn to make me worried, as they suggest a third reason to be concerned about medical marijuana. It's a reason that's both
intriguing and surprising. It's also one I'm embarrassed to admit that I
haven't thought of.

"Think about how people say marijuana helps them," Franklin says. "There's pain and nausea, sure. But people also use it for anxiety and panic attacks and insomnia, right?"

I nod, thinking about Tomas, but I'm not sure where this is going.

"And what are the symptoms of marijuana withdrawal?" she asks, leaning over her desk toward me.

Well, anxiety, panic attacks, insomnia . . . But I'm still not following. Goldman helps me out.

"The reasons that people say marijuana helps them are also some of the most prominent symptoms of marijuana withdrawal," she suggests. "You use, then you don't, and you start having low-grade withdrawal symptoms, so . . ."

"You use again," Franklin adds. "And you feel better."

They're suggesting that some of the psychological benefits that patients like Tomas perceive might not be benefits at all. That is, they're not necessarily experiencing less anxiety, for instance, than they did when they started using marijuana. It's just that they've gotten on a gentle roller-coaster ride in which their symptoms increase and decrease.

So Tomas would feel anxious, and he'd take a couple of hits, and he'd feel better. Then he'd stop using, and he'd experience symptoms of withdrawal that he interpreted as anxiety. Then he'd use again. And maybe each subsequent use made him a little more dependent, ensuring that he'd continue to have to self-medicate.

Indeed, in an enormous meta-analysis of 267 studies, researchers found an association between marijuana use and anxiety.[25] One interpretation of these results is exactly what Franklin and Goldman are suggesting. Maybe some of these regular marijuana users are experiencing chronic withdrawal symptoms, which manifest as anxiety.

But that's just one interpretation. It's also possible that people with chronic anxiety turn to marijuana to self-medicate. That might also produce the same association between marijuana use and anxiety that this study found.

I'd still like to think that Tomas finally found something that worked for him, without the side effects of all of the legal drugs he'd been prescribed. I'd like to think that even if he wasn't cured, he found something that he could use to make his symptoms manageable. But now I wonder.

Franklin walks me out, and I reflect on the crash course in the science of addiction I've just been through. In the past two hours, I've heard a pretty compelling case for the dangers of addiction.

That, by itself, doesn't worry me a lot. The risk of addiction shouldn't prompt an outright rejection of marijuana for medical purposes. Opioids like morphine, for instance, are addictive. And yet they're a legal and essential part of our armamentarium for treating pain. So I'm comfortable with that.

But what bothers me more is the fact that medical marijuana doesn't come with the restrictions that apply to opioids. For instance, as I'm about to discover, pretty much anyone can get medical marijuana. That lack of control makes for a potentially ominous future if medical marijuana use becomes widespread.

"It has the potential to become an epidemic," Franklin tells me as we say good-bye.

You could say her final warning to me sounds like fearmongering. And a few hours ago, I would have laughed it off. But knowing that there is an "addiction circuit" makes it impossible for me to dismiss concerns about marijuana addiction. A picture really is worth a thousand words, and that picture of a brain lighting up in anticipation is scary. So now the threat of addiction seems like something we need to take seriously.

The Marijuana Club

I'm convinced of the addictive potential of marijuana, but I'd like another perspective on the difference between medical and recreational users. The patients I'm meeting are getting a physician's recommendation and going to legal dispensaries, rather than buying dime bags on a street corner. Surely that's a relevant difference? To find out, I look up a researcher who has become fascinated by marijuana dispensaries and how people use them.

Steve Lankenau looks like a college student who has aged gracefully into the university faculty. He's tall and thin, with long, dark hair that he wears swept back. That, plus the cords and V-neck sweater worn over a T-shirt, make him look like the consummately cool teacher. It helps, I'm sure, that the topic he studies—marijuana use—is sure to be appealing to the entire undergraduate student body. He ushers me into his immaculate office, with shelves full of social science titles, many of which I remember scratching my head over in college.

Lankenau isn't a doctor or a biologist, and he's not interested in the science of medical marijuana. Or, at most, he's peripherally interested. He's a sociologist, and he's investigating the culture of medical marijuana use.

He's doing a large study of the ways in which young adults use medical marijuana. He's really interested in how medical use is different from recreational use. And he has an idea I want to learn about.

Lankenau thinks that the dynamics of addiction may be different when people get marijuana from a dispensary as opposed to on the street. Specifically, he thinks their risk of addiction, and progression to harder drugs, might be lower than it is for recreational users, for two reasons.

First, he thinks that clinics and dispensaries might reduce the risk of addiction.

"There's a range of clinics," he says. "Some are just transactional." He means you go in with a specific task in mind. Getting a marijuana recommendation is like buying a tankful of gas or getting a manicure. You know what you want, you get what you need, and you're out the door.

"But a lot of clinics and dispensaries are relational." He means that relationships develop, and those relationships define what takes place. So it's not simply a matter of getting what you want, but working with dispensary staff to figure out what you need.

Lankenau thinks that those relationships might help to reduce the risk of addiction. Relationships create feedback loops, for instance, about appropriate use. They offer nudges for people who are using too much, or letting their work or relationships suffer. And they provide moral support, too.

He knows enough about the risks of addiction not to be cavalier about them. But he thinks it's possible that the clinic and dispensary environment might protect medical marijuana users from addiction, at least partly. Sure, the biology of addiction might be the same wherever—and however—someone is using marijuana. But the support that people get through these clinics might help to dull those biological effects, avoiding some of the worst manifestations of addiction.

There's another reason Lankenau thinks that clinics and dispensaries might be protective, but it doesn't have anything to do with addiction to marijuana per se.

"The gateway theory of addiction," he tells me, "says that a slide into addiction often starts with one drug. People use that drug, but then they want more. More of an effect. Or a different effect. Variety. Something new."

Indeed, in one study of more than six thousand people whose first drug was marijuana, about 45 percent went on to use another illegal drug.[26] So, Lankenau says, they usually move on to cocaine or heroin or methamphetamine. In addition to whatever addictive potential marijuana itself has, according to this theory, it also brings with it a "downstream" risk of addiction to harder drugs.

"That craving for variety might lead to harder drugs if someone buys marijuana on the street. But dispensaries have endless choices. You've got lots of strains and potencies and mixes of THC and CBD. And of course there are edibles."

Lankenau thinks that the wide variety of products that are available in a typical dispensary could fulfill desires for something new and different. And that, in turn, might keep medical marijuana users from moving on to the next drug. Instead of trying cocaine, for instance, a marijuana user might try a different marijuana strain. Or a water pipe, or a vaporizer. That would be a much safer way to satisfy the desire for variety.

All this is speculative, of course. Even the study that Lankenau is doing won't provide definitive answers. But if he's right, and if medical use is different—and maybe safer—then I'll be a little less worried about the concerns that Franklin and Goldman have raised.

That doesn't mean that marijuana isn't addictive. It certainly is, and withdrawal is real. But I'm a little less worried about how people like Tomas and Alice and Rachel are doing, and whether they're going to get into trouble down the road.

Weed and Wheels

I admit that I was initially skeptical about the psychiatric risks of marijuana, and the likelihood of addiction. However, there is another risk that I was convinced was real. Indeed, this is a risk that I figured was pretty obvious: driving while under the influence.

That just seems like a really bad idea. Just how bad an idea it is, though, will require some research. And that's why I'm standing in the middle of a parking lot with one of my patients.

"If you think we're about to hit a tree or something," Jeff says, "just poke me, OK?"

It's at this point that I realize I'm embarking on the strangest patient visit I've ever done in my career as a doctor.

Jeff and I are standing next to his car in the parking lot of a middle school in suburban Philadelphia on a Saturday morning. And Jeff is stoned. I know this because in the past two minutes I've watched him demolish an entire joint of what he assures me is "really sweet" medical-grade marijuana. It was a gift, he tells me cheerfully, from a friend in California.

He drops the butt on the pavement and grinds it under his heel with a surprising degree of meticulousness. Then, carefully, he opens the door and slides into the driver's seat. With more than a little trepidation, I climb into the passenger seat. Things are about to get strange.

We're here to evaluate the effect of marijuana on Jeff's driving ability.

The car we're sitting in is an elderly Honda Civic, whose chassis has pretty much succumbed to a decade of Philadelphia winters. That wear has created a few gaps through which the outside world is visible. Jeff looks about as worn out as his car. He's been through a lot, too.

Jeff is in his forties, with neat, sandy hair that looks like it's been trimmed fresh this morning. He's wearing geeky black-framed glasses, and usually dresses carefully in khakis and oxford shirts that are worn and frayed, yet neatly pressed and ironed.

He used to be a manager in a loan financing company, a single parent of a teenage son, with a house in the suburbs. But then he started to suffer flashes of pain that would come on suddenly, engulfing the lower half of his body. He told me that during these episodes he felt like he was being dipped in liquid electricity. The pain led to an opioid addiction and then to the loss of his job.

Eventually his doctors discovered he had a slow-growing spinal tumor called a meningioma. With that diagnosis, Jeff was able to get better pain management that let him hold down a clerical job. And he could maintain some semblance of a normal life for his son Charlie as he made plans for surgery that he'll undergo this summer, when Charlie can go stay with his grandparents while Jeff is in rehab.

He just needs to manage his pain until summer, which is six months away. That's why he started using marijuana. At a clinic appointment with me a month ago, he mentioned that marijuana seemed to help his pain. He was also sleeping better when he used it at night. It worked so well, in fact, that he started using during the day. That's when he told me that he'd just smoked half a joint two hours ago.

There was a long pause in our conversation as I glanced at my watch—9:30 a.m.—and as I thought about the fact that Jeff lived in a suburb about fifteen miles away.

And so how did he get to the clinic?

"I drove."

There was an even longer pause.

"It's just a straight shot on I-76," he reassured me. "After I dropped Charlie off at school."

It began to dawn on me that Jeff's meningioma was not necessarily the greatest threat to his health. And other commuters in the Philadelphia metropolitan area should be very, very concerned.

I asked him then if he was OK with driving.

"Oh, sure. I do it all the time. I have to. Charlie needs to get to school, and I need to get to work. That's not a problem, is it?"

Was it? I wasn't sure. My gut feeling was that, yes, in fact, it was a problem. A big 65-mile-per-hour problem.

But really? I had no idea. I'd always thought that being high while driving was as dangerous as being drunk. Something you shouldn't do, ever.

But I also had to admit to Jeff that I didn't know. They don't teach you that kind of thing in medical school. Any training I've had about marijuana and driving could be summarized in a single word: Don't.

As a compromise, when we wrapped up that visit, we agreed to some ground rules. First, that Jeff wouldn't smoke within six hours of getting behind the wheel. (That six-hour rule, by the way, was a guess. I had no idea what a safe interval might be. But more about this later.) Second, he'd try to stick to backstreets whenever possible.

I also promised him I'd do some research, and later I turned up a couple of studies that seemed to offer a stern warning against driving while stoned. For instance, one large review compiled nine studies. Those studies used a variety of different methods, but the overall conclusion was that marijuana makes an accident about two and a half times more likely than when you're sober.[27] Another review I found also included nine studies, some of which were the same. That review found an approximately twofold increase in the risk of accidents.[28] Taken together, these results are pretty compelling that marijuana and driving don't mix.

Incidentally, these risks aren't limited to drivers in cars. If you're too stoned to drive, don't hop on a bicycle instead. That's the message of a study of bicycle accidents that found that the risk of riders' impairment when stoned is about the same as it is when drunk.[29]

Those studies are all worrisome, but there was also the fact that Jeff hasn't yet had an accident. That didn't make sense, given how much he was smoking. And so, puzzled, I proposed today's experiment.

The Banana Obstacle Course

We're both curious about marijuana's effects on Jeff's driving. And I'm curious about his insight. If he's impaired, can he recognize that he's a danger to others?

Jeff suggested this parking lot because he figured it would be empty on a Saturday. The only nearby obstacles are the ones that I've provided.

I envisioned performing this test with traffic cones, but alas, I didn't plan ahead. And buying two dozen traffic cones on a Saturday morning proved to be impossible. So instead I stopped at a grocery store and picked up ten pounds of bananas, leaving behind a bemused cashier. As Jeff was turning his joint to ashes, I arranged twenty-four bananas in two parallel lines, about ten feet apart, with about twelve feet between each line.

As we sit in Jeff's car I explain my plan. First, he'll drive between the two lines of bananas. Then he'll back up the same way. Then, as fast as he can, he's going to weave through the bananas on the right side, execute a U-turn, and then weave through the other line.

It's a simple plan, and Jeff is nodding. But it seems like he's paying a little too much attention to a flock of seagulls clustered at the far end of the parking lot. I'm not sure he's getting this. Banana carnage is a near certainty. I tighten my seat belt.

But Jeff isn't ready to drive. He's not quite sure where to put his feet. He admits he usually doesn't get behind the wheel so soon after smoking. So we sit in companionable silence while Jeff watches the parking lot's resident seagulls.

How long are we going to have to wait until Jeff's brain rejoins us? Based on what I've read in the executive report on marijuana and driving that was published by the National Highway Traffic Safety Administration, it might be some time.[30] That document is about as dull as it sounds, perhaps because the clean-living folks at the NHTSA are not terribly enthusiastic about drivers getting stoned. Their warnings are correspondingly strict.

They suggest, first, that marijuana impairs driving ability immediately. They also warn that its effects can last for up to three hours, and that residual effects can be seen for up to twenty-four hours. That's a pretty wide window, and twenty-four hours is a long time to be sitting in a parked car in the dead of winter.

If you look at studies of blood levels, the truth that emerges is a little more reassuring. It turns out that when you smoke marijuana, the two psychoactive substances that appear in the blood do so at different times. First, there's THC. That peaks in the bloodstream as people are smoking. The peaks, in fact, correspond to the timing and volume of an intake of breath.

So as Jeff was sucking down that joint a few minutes ago, his THC levels probably looked a little like the edge of a saw: up-down-up-down. But the baseline of that wave increases over time as the joint disappears. Imagine that jagged saw edge propped at a 45-degree angle and you have a pretty good idea of what's been happening in Jeff's brain. The net result is that his THC concentrations reached a peak in the minutes after finishing that joint.

Soon, however, those concentrations will subside. That's the good news. But that doesn't mean that in a few minutes he'll figure out where to put his feet.

Remember that THC is metabolized to 11-hydroxy-THC, which is as potent as THC, but has a longer half-life in the bloodstream. Its peak concentrations hit between ten to twenty minutes after smoking. (CBD appears in the blood, too, but as we've seen, it doesn't seem to have any effect on thinking or driving.)

Twenty minutes after Jeff finished his joint he says he feels a little better. Yet he looks about the same, and indeed he's still staring straight ahead, smiling, and laughing occasionally. So I'm eager to see what "better" looks like once our wheels start turning.

First, Jeff seems to rediscover his feet, and he puts the car in gear.

The concept of a manual transmission seems gloriously fresh to him. He contemplates the gearshift with intense satisfaction and chuckles as if it's telling him a joke he's heard several times before. After a juddering stall, Jeff restarts the aged Civic and repeats this maneuver. This time he also releases the parking brake.

The forward trip between the bananas goes well at first. We're about halfway down the corridor, traveling at a blistering five miles an hour, according to the Civic's tremulous speedometer, when we begin to veer subtly but unmistakably to the right. I can't hear the next banana meet its maker as it disappears under the right front tire, but a quick glance in the rearview mirror reveals that what remains is not pretty. I wonder what students and teachers are going to think when they arrive on Monday morning.

Then Jeff corrects our course, swinging the car a little too forcefully back toward the midline. He overcorrects, so that we're cruising toward the last banana on the left side. Closer . . . closer . . . Then it, too, becomes another stain on the pavement.

Marijuana studies conducted in driving simulators confirm that Jeff is exhibiting the classic behavior of someone driving while stoned. Interestingly, there have also been studies in flight simulators, although it's not clear to me why anyone thought that mixing marijuana with high altitude might be even remotely acceptable.[31] Jeff's sea-level performance in this empty parking lot is plenty scary enough for me.

There's no doubt, in fact, from years of such experiments—in virtual cars and planes—that marijuana is dangerous. In one such study, twenty-four volunteers were randomized to get a dose of THC or a placebo. Then researchers tracked how well the subjects stayed on the virtual road. They found that the THC subjects did much worse, and had a much harder time steering in a straight line. They also found that the THC subjects were much slower in adjusting their speed to avoid the car in front of them.[32] Of particular interest, a similar study recruited both occasional and chronic marijuana users and found that with the same dose, chronic users performed worse, which suggests that there might be a cumulative effect that builds over time.[33] In light of Jeff's use over the past couple of months, this is not good news for those bananas still intact.

There's another feature of Jeff's motoring behavior that also appears in simulators, but it's one that's a little counterintuitive. Specifically, he's not doing as badly as he should be. This is a guy who, just a few minutes ago, couldn't find his feet. And yet he's able to shift gears and keep the car (more or less) on track. That is, he's able to compensate.

Although his driving is certainly impaired, and although I'd estimate his chances of murdering a tree as being at least ten times what it was in his sober state, he's not flattened. He's functioning—sort of.

In general, stoned drivers seem to recognize, at some level, that they're a few neurons short of a full brain. They know that they're impaired, and they adapt. They slow down, for instance. Jeff certainly did.

And that's good news. Going slowly gives stoned drivers a wider margin of error. Jeff's reaction times are probably pretty sluggish, but if he's driving slowly enough, that provides a few extra milliseconds for his brain to catch up with events. Enough, maybe, to spare a banana or two.

Jeff has something else going for him. He's a naturally cautious guy and—I'm guessing—a cautious driver. In a study of seventy-two people in a driving simulator, test subjects who had driven while using marijuana in the past had a more aggressive driving style when sober.[34] That raises the interesting possibility that at least some of the association between marijuana use and accidents might be due to personality. Although marijuana certainly impairs driving, it's also possible that at least some accidents happen because the guy behind the wheel is just reckless. And Jeff certainly isn't.

As he reaches the end of the obstacle course, he comes to a gradual stop. I remind him that the next task is to back up through the gauntlet that he'd just run. He nods, concentrating fiercely on his rearview mirror.

Again he puts the car into gear, and I notice that we're barely moving. We're going so slowly that Jeff is having trouble preventing the car from stalling. As he turns his attention from the rearview mirror to focus on the delicate work of moving his right foot on the gas pedal, we veer to the left and clip another banana. This happens two more times during the short course, and three more bananas die on this run. (The total body count, in case you're keeping score, is five bananas. And we aren't nearly done.)

There's a lesson here, too. It turns out that whether marijuana has a substantial effect on driving depends on what else is going on. When driving tasks are relatively simple (stop, go, turn), stoned drivers do OK, because they go slowly. Not great, but OK. And in simulations they usually manage to avoid killing or maiming anyone.

But when things start getting complicated, driving performance plummets. If speed increases, as it does on a highway, then reaction times can't keep up. Or if a driver faces multiple tasks (changing gears, switching lanes, navigating), performance goes to hell pretty quickly.

This gets interesting if you look inside a brain that's stoned using functional magnetic resonance imaging. One fascinating fMRI study of thirty-one male volunteers found that marijuana use produces three main changes in drivers' brains.[35] First, the researchers found that stoned brain activity was decreased in several areas of the brain, including the dorsomedial thalamus.

Changes there are correlated with what psychologists describe in their typically poetic way as "salience detection." Put simply, this is our ability to focus. So sensory perceptions of pretty clouds, and the slap of the windshield wipers, and the flow of air over your hand that's hanging out the window compete for attention with the bumper of the car in front of you that's getting a bit too close.

The same study found a similar decrease in activity in the brain's right superior parietal cortex and in the dorsolateral prefrontal cortex. Those changes suggest a decrease in executive function, or the ability to figure out what's important, to prioritize. So to a stoned brain, not only are those clouds pretty, they're as important as the stop sign . . . that you just passed.

Third, that fMRI study revealed an increase in activity in the brain's cortex—the outer layer that's related to higher thought and motor function. Specifically, the researchers found an increase in the rostral anterior cingulate cortex and ventromedial prefrontal cortex. This is particularly interesting, because it reflects a focus on internal thoughts and sensations. In effect, this increase in activity reflects an increased introspective focus on "me" to the exclusion of the surrounding world. Thinking about yourself is fine, of course. But there's a time and a place for introspection, and a crowded Philadelphia street isn't it.

How Stoned Is Too Stoned?

There's a rather large question hovering in the background of all of this discussion of brain imaging. It's one thing to say that marijuana and driving don't mix. Fair enough. I'd be happy to give that rule a hearty endorsement.

However, that wasn't what Jeff asked me. He didn't want to know whether marijuana impaired his driving. He wanted to know how to use marijuana and still drive safely. And this experiment hasn't given us an answer yet.

It would be nice if Jeff had some way of figuring out whether he was too stoned to drive. The equivalent of a breathalyzer test for alcohol. But what?

Unfortunately, there isn't currently such a test that works. THC is probably responsible for marijuana's impact on driving, but THC levels don't correlate well with driving performance. In that same fMRI study I mentioned earlier, blood levels weren't associated with fMRI changes, either. That is, people with higher THC blood levels didn't show more brain effects. So a simple test of your THC blood levels won't help you figure out whether or not you can get behind the wheel of a car.

But there's another test we could use, right now. I describe it to Jeff. He seems wryly amused, then laughs and agrees to try it.

Following my instructions, Jeff gets out of the car and faces the empty parking lot. He tilts his head lightly back and stretches his arms out wide, as if he's about to join the flock of seagulls circling over the distant soccer field. Then he closes his eyes.

Agonizingly slowly, Jeff brings his right forefinger within range of his nose, and then he drops it for a perfect landing. He opens his eyes and grins, as if this is a prize-worthy achievement.

Then Jeff repeats this amazing feat with his left finger. A little more quickly this time, with a concomitant loss of accuracy. Still, his forefinger manages to touch down on his nose. More or less.

We try a few other sobriety test maneuvers, like standing on one leg, and walking along one of the white parking space lines. Despite his current THC levels, and despite his meningioma, which is probably limiting him at least a little, Jeff does quite well. Perhaps he's a little slower than a sober person would be. But he definitely passes.

Indeed, it turns out that the classic "field sobriety test" that's used to detect alcohol intoxication is pretty useless for identifying drivers who are stoned. In one study of chronic users, volunteers were given about 25 milligrams of THC (more or less, depending on their weight). That THC didn't seem to impair the volunteers' ability to touch their noses, although they were slightly more unsteady when asked to stand on one leg.[36]

But the same group of researchers did another study. This time, they didn't want to know whether THC affected performance, but whether either the finger-to-nose test or the standing test was able to distinguish between volunteers who had received THC and those who hadn't. It didn't distinguish. A coin flip would have provided a more accurate test.

So how does a marijuana user like Jeff determine if he or she is likely to get in trouble on the road? He can't rely on a test like a breathalyzer to detect THC levels. And standing on one leg or touching his nose isn't a useful test, either. So then, what?

There's a pretty simple answer, although it's not going to assuage the concerns of many state troopers. In that fMRI study of stoned drivers, although fMRI changes weren't associated with blood levels of THC, there was a strong correlation with feelings of confusion. That is, the subjective feeling of confusion was a good predictor of MRI changes.

So a good test of driving ability might be as simple as an honest self-assessment. Maybe the best predictor of whether your drive to the grocery store is going to end in a collision with a tree is how stoned you feel.

I decide to try this out on Jeff who, remember, has just smashed five bananas and passed a field sobriety test. I mention that we still have one more segment of the test to go, in which he'll weave along one line of bananas, execute a U-turn, and then weave through the other line. How well does he think he'll do?

"Oh . . . not too good?"

I'll second that. Score one for self-assessment. But for the sake of science we need to finish the test, so we climb back into Jeff's car and I buckle up.

The weaving segment of my improvised course is, alas, something of a letdown. Only three more bananas are crushed, bringing the grand total to eight. That's the good news. The bad news is that it takes Jeff almost ten painfully slow minutes to drive 120 feet, turn around, and drive back.

As Jeff brings the car to a stop, he seems to be aware of his performance.

"I didn't do too well, did I?"

He's right—he didn't. Of twenty-four bananas that began this adventure, eight have been reduced to the consistency of baby food. It's amazing, in fact, how closely our little experiment was consistent with the scientific literature. Jeff was distracted, and cautious, and he overcompensated.

And yet Jeff doesn't seem to care that he just failed a pitifully easy test in much the same condition that he's driven on I-76. It's as if we're talking about someone else's performance. Someone whose travels would not bring him within a thousand miles of his son Charlie or anyone else Jeff cares about.

We agree to the rules that I'd suggested earlier: Before driving anywhere, wait at least six hours, and then stick to backstreets. And, just for good measure, I add the self-assessment rule. If he thinks he can't drive, or if Charlie thinks he's impaired, he shouldn't get behind the wheel. I'm not entirely comfortable with that plan. But I'm pretty sure anything stricter wouldn't hold up.

There's one more question I need to ask Jeff, though. How is he going to get home?

"I live just up that street over there—about ten blocks."

And...?

"Can I get a ride?"

Keep Off the Grass?

It's difficult to know what to make of all of these risks. On one hand, there's some compelling evidence that we should take them seriously. Add to that the fact that many of these risks—psychosis, brain damage, schizophrenia—are intuitively obvious. It's easy to see how the short-term effect of marijuana, such as hallucinations and disordered thinking, could lead to long-term problems.

On the other hand, just because risks are intuitively obvious doesn't mean they're legitimate. Indeed, their obviousness seems to incite opponents of marijuana to make dire warnings. Some of the most vociferous fearmongering I've heard has been about these psychiatric risks.

Nevertheless, there are some risks we need to worry about if we're going to prescribe marijuana as medicine. Here's my best attempt at a summary.

First, psychosis and schizophrenia. To me, the evidence of a link between marijuana use and psychosis is pretty persuasive. In fact, I'd probably go so far as to say that anyone with a previous history of a psychotic episode should probably stay away from the stuff. And—what will probably not endear me to medical marijuana advocates—I'd probably also at least want to warn other patients who have one or more risk factors, such as a family history of schizophrenia, substance abuse, disordered thinking, or paranoia.

However, even if Tomas had these risk factors, I wouldn't tell him outright that he shouldn't use medical marijuana. It's ultimately his choice. Besides, that would be a pretty tough message to deliver, since marijuana is the only thing he's found that's helped him. But he deserves to know about the risks he might be facing so that he can make an informed decision.

As for the risk of schizophrenia, that evidence seems less persuasive. It's certainly possible that there is a link between marijuana use and schizophrenia. Indeed, if you believe that there's a link with psychosis, and if psychosis and schizophrenia are similar, it stands to reason that marijuana users are at increased risk of schizophrenia, too. But based solely on the studies I've found, I don't think we can make that case yet.

The evidence for brain damage due to long-term use is even more speculative. Sure, there have been some studies that have found long-term effects, but others haven't. And we really don't understand how subtle changes in the brain's structure affect thinking, which is what we really care about.

There's a caveat here, though, and it's an important one. Whether a possible risk of brain damage matters will depend a lot on the person. Earlier I described the brain as a call center, with reserves that get called up as we need them. Well, if cognitive function, the clearest head possible, is really important to you—for your work or your life—then you'll want to make sure those reserves are in good shape. And you should probably be more wary of taking any risks.

Granted, a joint now and again probably won't limit your ability to do *The New York Times* crossword puzzle twenty years from now. But regular use could have that effect. And if that possibility scares you—even though it's only a possibility—you might want to curb your use.

The risk of addiction is easier to summarize. After spending an afternoon with Franklin and Goldman and their screens full of glowing brains, I'm about as certain as I can be that marijuana really is addictive. And marijuana withdrawal is a real concern.

True, we use other addictive drugs in medicine, so the potential for addiction shouldn't disqualify marijuana for medical use. But when people use drugs like morphine for chronic conditions, they generally know that those pills may be habit forming, and they have physicians who have prescribed the pills and should be monitoring their use. Right now, that careful attention and oversight doesn't exist for medical marijuana. So anyone using marijuana for medical use is going to need to understand the risks of addiction and watch for the signs of addiction, including tolerance, withdrawal, and interference with their lives.

Finally, if you're thinking of getting high and then driving a car or operating heavy machinery, or flying a plane, that's easy. Don't. Just don't.

7

Bodily Harm

Perhaps you were as surprised as I was to learn about the psychological risks of marijuana. If so, you may be dismayed to learn that its risks aren't limited to the brain. In fact, there are a lot of potential risks that have nothing to do with psychiatric illness or addiction. There are reported risks of physical side effects—bronchitis, lung disease, and lung cancer, for instance. Strokes, too. And heart attacks.

That list is disturbing, especially if you happen to be a user of marijuana yourself. But don't panic.

Although some risks are real, others are pretty clearly the product of fearmongering. Still others—and this is the big challenge—we just don't know enough about.

In this chapter, I'll describe the most likely risks, and I'll introduce you to research and researchers who can put those risks in perspective. I'll also take you to a testing laboratory that's trying to protect medical marijuana users by giving them reliable information about the ingredients of whatever they're smoking.

This chapter is full of surprises. At least, researching it was often surprising for me. Some risks that I'd taken for granted, such as lung damage, turn out to be much less of a problem than I'd imagined. And other risks that I'd never thought of, such as a disappearing penis, seem to be all too real.

Pulmonary Function Testing Smackdown

You'd think that smoking marijuana would cause lung damage, right? You're burning and inhaling plant matter and—according to Steve, the guy who introduced me to his Volcano—insect legs. That can't be a good thing. Especially since we know that smoking cigarettes causes lung damage, logically marijuana should, too.

But does it? In every chapter of this book so far, I've been surprised by things about marijuana that I didn't know, so I don't want to assume that smoking marijuana is bad for your lungs. I want to find out.

That's why I'm in a small, bare, windowless room, accompanied by a fit young man named James. He's got a high-and-tight buzz cut and is wearing hospital scrubs and running shoes.

James ushers me into a box that looks like a short, fat, transparent phone booth. It's a metal frame that has Plexiglas walls on all four sides, plus the roof, which yields a spectacular view of a particleboard ceiling. There's a plastic seat against one wall and a white plastic tube protruding from the opposite wall. There is also, disturbingly, what looks like a latch on the outside of the door.

"It's hermetically sealed," James says helpfully. "Airtight."

I've agreed to be locked in an airtight booth because I want to get a firsthand look at how my lung function compares to that of one of my patients. Marijuana smoking is measured in terms of joint-years, and my patient, Chris, has smoked a joint every day for about twenty years, or twenty joint-years. That's a lot, so when he told me that he felt like he didn't have the exercise tolerance that he used to, I sent him for pulmonary function testing.

In order to understand the effects of that much smoking on a pair of lungs, we need the pulmonary function tests of someone who doesn't have twenty joint-years of experience with marijuana. We also need someone of about the same age. So here I am.

I sit down, and James moves a tube—which is mounted on an intricate hinged contraption—up and to the left, so it hovers at mouth level.

"Your mouth is going to go all the way around that," he says.

James gives me a chance to get used to breathing through what feels like a large, complicated snorkel. There's just the tiniest bit of resistance—just a little pop at first as a valve opens. Then he puts a plastic clamp on my nose.

"OK?"

Ummm, I guess. Thus encumbered, I can't nod. So I try a thumbs-up sign. This seems to reassure James.

"Start out breathing normally."

I do.

"Now big breath in . . . OK . . . and blow blow blow blow blow harder harder harder."

I breathe. Then I blow.

"Now a big breath in really fast."

I breathe.

Next, James closes and latches the door. I can hear his voice through a speaker in front of me. His instructions echo in the small space, making it sound like we're underwater. He gives me more instructions that involve deep breaths, shallow breaths, panting, and more deep breaths. In one maneuver, he has me put my hands on my cheeks and pant into the tube. I imagine I probably look like a bong-smoking version of Edvard Munch's painting *The Scream*.

Finally, James opens the door, and I remove mouth from tube and clip from nose. That wasn't so bad. I thank James and make my way to the hospital cafeteria. I figure this is as good a place as any to review my results and Chris's. Who won?

Waiting for my espresso, I have ample time to try to recall what I learned long ago in medical school about pulmonary function tests. One measurement is total lung capacity, which is pretty much what it sounds like. It's how much air you can hold in your lungs in a maximal breath, plus what's left over in your lungs after you exhale. In the test I just experienced, that was calculated by my deep breath in. (It's more complicated than that, but you get the idea.)

Another measurement is the forced expiratory volume at one second (FEV1), which is the amount of air in your lungs that you can exhale in one second. That was the blow-blow-blow-blow part. The FEV1 is reduced in longtime tobacco smokers because their lungs become weak and baggy. As that happens, the act of trying to force air out of the lungs closes off airways, increasing airway resistance and reducing airflow.

There's also the forced vital capacity (FVC). That's how much air you can move in and out of your lungs. This measurement is usually increased a little in chronic smokers because those baggy lungs have gotten bigger over time. They don't work as well, but they hold more air.

There are many other measurements, but those are the main ones, the measurements we want to focus on to understand the long-term effects of marijuana smoking.

So how did Chris do? And how did I do? And—most important for my pulmonary ego—did I beat him?

I take a seat in the cafeteria with both our test results spread out in front of me. Because normal values depend on a person's size, I look to the far right of our reports, which display our numbers as a percent of what would be normal for people with our dimensions.

First, our FEV1s. Mine is 98 percent of normal and Chris's is 99 percent. Given the variation in a normal population, that means we're both normal. So far so good, for both of us.

Second, our vital capacities are normal, too. Mine, again, is 98 percent. His is 105 percent. His total lung capacity is also higher than mine. Technically he and I are both "normal." But his lungs can hold more air than mine can, after adjusting for our sizes.

I'm trying not to take that result personally. How could a professional-grade marijuana smoker do as well, or even a little better, than a relatively young, fit doctor (who isn't a smoker)? This doesn't seem fair.

I'm miffed. I'm also confused. So I decide to pay a visit to the person who is best able to explain this injustice.

The Pulmonary Soothsayer

I'm standing in the lobby of the Ronald Reagan UCLA Medical Center in Los Angeles looking for Dr. Donald Tashkin, a pulmonary physician who specializes in tests of lung function, like the ones that Chris and I underwent. And this guy is good.

He doesn't just interpret the present—he predicts the future. He can look at your test results and tell you whether in twenty years you'll be able to run a marathon or whether you'll be tethered to an oxygen tank. I'm here because a lot of Tashkin's studies have included people with more than a passing familiarity with marijuana.[1] If anyone knows what marijuana could do to the lungs—now and in twenty years—it's him.

But where is he?

Then I see someone who must be the guy I'm looking for. He's small and lean, with a noticeable list to starboard. He has close-cropped white hair and wire frame glasses, and he's impeccably dressed in a snow-white lab coat that seems to illuminate our corner of the lobby as he walks in.

Courtly and polite, he's walked across the UCLA campus to meet me, warning that I'd never find my way. He suggests we find a place to sit and talk nearby, and I feel bad that this frail, older man has journeyed a quarter of a mile for my sake. It must have been difficult for him.

But then Tashkin launches himself in the direction of the cafeteria with strides that are so rapid that I have trouble keeping up. As we fly through the lobby and down one hall after another, he inquires about my trip, and my stay in Los Angeles, and whether I'd like coffee. Obviously his pulmonary function is hunky-dory. I'm no longer so confident about mine.

Finally, we reach the hospital cafeteria and take seats on opposite sides of a long, empty table. I take a couple of deep breaths. After looking me over with what seems like professional concern, Tashkin begins talking.

Over a fascinating couple of hours, he walks me through the history of research into the pulmonary effects of marijuana with the sure-footedness of a lecturer who has been over this territory a million times.

First, Tashkin tells me about lung damage. "The evidence is clear that tobacco smoke causes COPD," he reminds me. (COPD is chronic obstructive pulmonary disease, or emphysema.) "There's no doubt about that whatsoever. Tobacco smoke accelerates the loss in lung function that we see with aging."

He explains that marijuana smoke contains many of the same chemicals that are present in tobacco smoke, like phenols, aldehydes, oxides of nitrogen, as well as tar and particulates (like bits of burnt insect legs). It's a long list that includes a lot of things that can cause inflammation and eventual lung damage. However, most studies haven't found that marijuana smoke causes lung damage. "In my research career," Tashkin says, "I've encountered two big surprises. This was one of them." (We'll get to the second in a little bit.)

Tashkin describes a large study that he and colleagues conducted involving 394 people. Some had smoked tobacco, others smoked marijuana, and some didn't smoke either. Much to Tashkin's surprise, he didn't find any evidence of lung damage in the marijuana group.[2]

That's pretty much the same conclusion of several other studies that have followed people for up to twenty years. One found no evidence of lung damage.[3] Another didn't, either, except for a slight reduction in FEV1 among heavy users, and an increase in FVC, the total amount of air you can breathe in and out).[4]

How could that be? Tashkin has a theory. He thinks that cannabinoids like THC and CBD have anti-inflammatory properties. And since a lot of the damage caused by smoke is due to inflammation, it's possible that cannabinoids protect against the damage that marijuana smoke is causing.

That's an intriguing theory, but Tashkin suggests another that's more mundane. It's possible that studies haven't found the tobacco-like lung damage in marijuana smokers simply because the typical marijuana exposure is much, much lower than the usual tobacco dose. Chris's one joint per day would qualify him as a moderately heavy marijuana user. In contrast, with tobacco, it's not unusual for a smoker to burn through a pack of twenty cigarettes every day, or more.

Think for a moment about what sort of condition you'd be in if you smoked twenty joints in a day. Your lung function would be the least of your problems. So it makes sense that marijuana doesn't cause the lung damage that tobacco does, simply because the amount of marijuana smoke that most people are exposed to is so much lower.

Fair enough. I can understand why marijuana smoking may not be harmful, at least in typical exposures of one or two joints per day. But what about Chris's lung capacity? It's one thing to say that chronic marijuana smoking isn't harmful. What could explain the fact that he had a greater lung capacity than someone of his age and weight should have? And greater than mine, since I was the nonsmoking control in this experiment. (This kind of disparity was also one result of one of the studies I just mentioned.)

Tashkin's answer? Practice. He explains that when marijuana smokers take repeated large, deep breaths, they're conditioning their lungs to stretch. It's not unlike the exercises that breath-holding skin divers use to pack as much air as possible into their lungs for prolonged periods underwater.

That's not really a good thing, though, he reminds me. Bigger lung capacity doesn't necessarily help you. And there are risks of that "practice." For one, you increase your risk of a pneumothorax, or acute hole in the lung, commonly known as a collapsed lung, by taking the deepest breath you can and holding it the way that most marijuana smokers do.

So, there's cause for both reassurance and caution in interpreting all of these results. Reassurance, because studies seem to indicate that any pulmonary risks are minor, and probably only apply to long-term, heavy use.

But Tashkin offers a warning. "We know that some people are predisposed to develop COPD. So even though marijuana smoke might not produce lung damage in the average person, if you've got that predisposition, you could still be at risk."

And perhaps the most important risk factor is your current lung function. "Lung function declines at a predictable rate with age," he says. "We lose a little every year." If someone already has a decreased FEV1 now, for instance, then smoking tobacco or marijuana is going to leave them in worse shape than it would in someone whose lungs were fine. So, even if marijuana smoke in moderate doses won't cause significant damage, if you're starting out with already existing damage due to tobacco smoke, you should probably be concerned about how much more damage your lungs will tolerate.

Goo and Cancer

All right, but what about more short-term effects of smoking? I'm thinking about studies that have found that marijuana smoking causes airway swelling and inflammation[5] and perhaps an increased risk of lung infections and chronic cough.[6] That makes sense to me. Smoke can't be good for our lungs. But then again, I was pretty sure that smoking marijuana would lead to chronic lung damage, and I was wrong. So I put this question to Tashkin.

"There's no doubt that marijuana smokers develop symptoms of bronchitis—that's a direct effect of the inflammation that the smoke causes." Even if cannabinoids reduce inflammation somewhat, all of the particulates and tar in marijuana overwhelm any protective effects.

This is the most emphatic assessment that Tashkin is willing to offer about any risk. "These effects are known."

Tashkin describes some of those effects in gory detail. For instance, there is an increase in inflammation and edema. There's also swelling in the layer of cells under the topmost epithelial layer.

"But the big problem is mucus."

Mucus?

Tashkin explains to me that it's all about the goo that lines our airways. "Smoke is an irritant. And that irritation causes destruction of ciliary cells." Those are the cells equipped with tiny brooms—cilia—that sweep particles of junk up out of our lungs. Those ciliary cells are replaced by goblet cells that secrete mucus. So with enough irritation, you get mucus. Often lots of it. With resultant coughing and disgusting phlegm.

"But," Tashkin says happily, "those symptoms are self-limited. When smokers stop, the symptoms resolve."

There's another effect of marijuana, though, that's astonishing to me. If the first surprise in Tashkin's career was his discovery that marijuana doesn't seem to cause long-term lung damage, the second is what he learned about marijuana's potential as therapy for asthma.

The idea of encouraging people with asthma to smoke sounds like a joke. But in the 1970s, Tashkin conducted a study along these lines. He explains he was initially interested in the acute effects of marijuana on the lung. He assumed that there would be acute changes like breathing difficulty. Or at least that he'd be able to document increased airway resistance and decreased airflow due to inflammation. But what he found was the opposite. Volunteers who smoked marijuana actually had better lung function immediately afterward.

He guessed that cannabinoids' anti-inflammatory effects might improve lung function. That could be useful, he knew, in conditions like asthma in which acute increases in inflammation increase airway resistance and decrease airflow. Indeed, Tashkin says that they tried marijuana in patients with asthma and found that their lung function actually improved. In fact, he says, he even worked with a colleague to put THC into a metered dose inhaler. I later found that in a small study of ten patients with asthma, inhaled THC did about as well as the drug salbutamol, a bronchodilator.[7] In theory, cannabinoids in edibles or tinctures might have the same effect, but Tashkin reasoned that the most efficient way to get a dose of cannabinoids into the lungs is to inhale them.

Those souped-up devices, sadly, never made it to clinical trials. I'm sure Tashkin's marijuana inhalers would have been wildly popular among people with asthma, and probably lots of other people.

At this point in our conversation, I'm feeling a little underwhelmed. I anticipated that Tashkin would give me a harsh and unsparing assessment of the risks of marijuana use. He is, after all, a lung doctor. I figured he'd be pretty critical. But so far, all I've heard is that bronchitis symptoms are a temporary effect. And that marijuana could be used to treat asthma. Seriously?

But I think I've got an ace in the hole. What about cancer? I'm thinking about lung cancer, of course. But also cancer in other locations that are exposed to marijuana smoke, such as the mouth and throat.

Tashkin nods. "Tobacco smoking is strongly associated with cancer in all of those sites. And the ingredients of tobacco smoke and marijuana smoke are pretty much identical."

I sense a "but" coming. And indeed there is.

He describes one of his studies that enrolled more than two thousand people and found no increased risk of cancer.[8] That study wasn't perfect, he admits. But it enrolled a large, diverse group of people, and really should have found an association if in fact one exists.

"The bottom line," Tashkin says, "is that there really isn't any good evidence of an increased risk of cancer." A more recent pooled analysis of approximately five thousand people also failed to find an association between marijuana use and lung cancer.[9]

The problem with these sorts of studies is that it's easy to be misled. One massive study of almost fifty thousand people found that marijuana use at a single point in time (during military enlistment) predicted a twofold increase risk of lung cancer.[10] However, although the researchers knew about tobacco smoking at that initial time point, they didn't know who began smoking tobacco later. If marijuana users were more likely to start smoking tobacco, then that cancer risk is probably due to tobacco, not to marijuana. But it's studies like this one, which enroll lots of people and follow them for a long time, that look impressive. They can be very convincing unless you read the fine print.

Of course, that doesn't mean that there isn't a risk. Maybe there is, but we just haven't found it. Nevertheless, from what we know right now, it seems safe to say that if there is a cancer risk of smoking marijuana, it's probably pretty small. And we really don't know whether there's a cancer risk of using marijuana in other forms.

Tashkin's phone has been buzzing more insistently for the past half hour. He's still as courtly and focused as he was when we met, offering references and citations for every point he makes, and pausing to make sure I'm getting names and dates right. But I have the sense that he has pressing obligations elsewhere.

"I have to go see a new patient," he admits, after checking his phone once again. "And I have a phone call in a few minutes."

I have one more question for him, though. And I hope it's an easy one. I've been thinking about these pulmonary risks, and about the increasing popularity of vaporizers. Wouldn't vaporizing eliminate these risks?

"Any risk would be from smoke inhalation. Smoke has carcinogens that are comparable to those in tobacco smoke. Carcinogens and oxidative stress. DNA damage. And particulates that can cause inflammation. You don't get those with cannabinoids in a vaporizer."

At all?

Tashkin shakes his head. "Nope."

In fact, in one small study of twelve heavy marijuana smokers, switching to a vaporizer improved their lung function and reduced goo-related symptoms.[11] So if you're still worried about what seem to be modest risks of smoking, you can dial your pulmonary risks down pretty close to zero with a vaporizer.

We say our good-byes, and Tashkin scoots across the cafeteria with amazing speed. A moment later he's gone, and I'm trying to catch up on my notes and to put everything that he's told me in perspective.

I have to admit that I'm more than a little surprised by what he's told me. But Tashkin seems pretty convinced that the big risks of COPD or cancer are really not much of a concern. And, as for the more modest risks of bronchitis, those seem to be self-limited and go away when users stop smoking.

Then there's also the intriguing possibility that vaporizing and other forms of ingestion might avoid even those risks. This would mean that even Rachel's use of a vape pen more than twenty times every day probably wasn't causing any significant lung damage. If the big concerns are related to smoke, and if you can get rid of that smoke . . . Well, marijuana is starting to sound pretty safe, at least for the lungs.

Hearts and Minds

Tashkin painted a pretty reassuring picture of marijuana effects on the lungs. Although there do seem to be some risks, they're much smaller than I thought they'd be. But what about other risks to the rest of the body?

There are some rather obvious short-term risks of marijuana use to the heart, like tachycardia (a fast heart rate). In a 1975 letter to the *New England Journal of Medicine*, a Dr. Schaefer advocated using the heart rate as a gauge for titrating marijuana dose in experiments "so that the rate can be accurately determined and, more importantly, so that smoking can be terminated as soon as the criterion heart-rate is reached."[12] No doubt the good Dr. Schaefer annoyed many of his research subjects by cutting them off as soon as their heart rate reached his own predetermined "criterion."

After a dose of marijuana, many patients also experience a drop in blood pressure when they stand up. That's known as orthostatic hypotension (orthostatic refers to standing upright, and hypotension is low blood pressure). When this happens, you might feel a little light-headed or dizzy. But it could be more of a problem in someone who is old or frail, and who might be predisposed to falls or fainting. Or in someone taking a blood thinner like warfarin, for whom a fall could result in internal bleeding. We don't know how big that risk is, though, because previous research has been done on recreational users who are generally young and healthy.

The combined increase in heart rate and drop in blood pressure could also be a concern for someone with heart disease. An increase in heart rate creates more work for the heart, and a drop in blood pressure means your heart isn't getting as much blood as it usually does. (The heart needs blood flow just like all of your other organs do.) So it's plausible that marijuana might cause more serious mischief, such as a heart attack, in someone who is predisposed. But does it?

In early studies, it seemed as though marijuana might actually cause heart attacks. At least, that was the worrisome conclusion of a study in which researchers interviewed people who had had a heart attack, and determined whether and when they'd last used marijuana. The researchers concluded that there was an approximately fivefold increase in heart attacks in the first hour after marijuana use.[13] That's probably enough to dissuade at least some people from ever touching a joint.

Added to those results is some evidence—at least in the laboratory—that THC induces platelets to coagulate (clot).[14] If you're bleeding from a cut, that's a good thing. But since we know that blood clotting in small vessels sets the stage for blocked coronary arteries, an enhanced ability to clot is potentially bad news for marijuana users.

Intrigued by their preliminary findings and these laboratory results, the researchers who found that fivefold increase in heart attack risk wanted to see whether marijuana use was associated with an increased risk of cardiac death. In a preliminary study of patients who had already suffered a heart attack, they followed patients for about four years, and they did find an increased risk.[15] The future of medical marijuana was looking tenuous indeed. Particularly for anyone with heart trouble. But in a later study, with up to eighteen years of follow-up, there was a trend, but no significant effect.[16]

So does marijuana increase the risk of a heart attack? Maybe. At least in the short term, an increase in heart rate and a drop in blood pressure might conceivably trigger a heart attack in someone who is predisposed. Longer-term risks don't seem to be a concern, but it's hard to say for sure. Nevertheless, people with a history of heart disease—and certainly those with a previous heart attack—should use marijuana with caution.

What about the brain? Strokes happen when a part of your brain isn't getting enough blood. So the same physiologic effects (decreased blood pressure and possibly increased blood clotting) that raise concerns about heart attacks could also cause strokes. Indeed, there have been case reports of strokes in marijuana users.[17] On the other hand, remember that in chapter 2 we saw that cannabinoids might have a protective effect in laboratory studies, limiting brain damage in mice after they've had a stroke.

Besides, these are just reports. There's no control group of people who used marijuana but didn't have a stroke. Look hard enough, and you can probably find examples of people having a stroke immediately after tying their shoes or eating strawberry ice cream. But that doesn't mean that either of these was responsible.

To figure out whether marijuana actually increases the risk of a stroke, we need a control group. One study found a control group in a novel way.[18] The researchers used a urine test to look for marijuana use in patients who had suffered a stroke, and also in normal controls, who had come to the emergency room for other reasons. They found that people who had just suffered a stroke were more likely to have used marijuana recently.

That's bad news at first glance, but it's not quite that simple. On further analysis, it turned out that this difference disappeared after adjusting for tobacco use. That is, the increased risk of stroke seemed to be explained by tobacco, not marijuana.

Undeterred, the authors nevertheless manage to wring a cautionary tale from these results: "This study provides evidence of an association between a cannabis lifestyle that includes tobacco and ischemic stroke." That seems like a bit of a stretch to me. It's a little like saying that baseball fans are more likely to chew tobacco, which causes mouth cancer, so therefore mouth cancer is associated with "the baseball fan lifestyle."

It's difficult to say that there's any clear association between marijuana use and strokes. Nevertheless, we do know a lot about the effects of marijuana on blood pressure and clotting. Therefore, it's probably smart to avoid marijuana use if you've had a stroke in the past, and particularly if you have other risk factors for a stroke, like high cholesterol, high blood pressure, or diabetes.

The Case of the Vanishing Penis and Other Risks of Marijuana

Even if the evidence that marijuana use affects the heart or brain is inconclusive, there are lots of other risks to worry about. Look hard enough, and you can find reports that marijuana causes all sorts of misery. I'll spare you most of them, but there are a few that stand out as being particularly relevant or interesting—or just plain weird.

In that last category, for instance, consider a study that recruited seventy-seven well-adjusted and otherwise apparently normal marijuana-using California college students and asked them about adverse reactions to marijuana.[19] Those college students described all of the usual side effects, including anxiety, hallucinations, and paranoia.

However, three men spontaneously reported that while they were high they developed the intense and unshakable belief that their penises were shrinking. What's really interesting is that these California college students were describing Koro. That's a culture-bound syndrome that has been described in Malaysia, China, and India, among other places. But not, until then, on a Los Angeles university campus among Caucasian students.

Fortunately, though, these penile difficulties seemed to be short-lived. One man reported that his organ returned to its normal contours after he took a bath. The second drank 12 ounces of wine and watched television for two hours, whereupon his penis reappeared. The third "took 5 mg of diazepam and drank two beers while watching cartoons."

The men apparently recovered with no aftereffects. Well, except for one.

"All three," the report concludes, "decreased their cannabis consumption after the Koro experience."

I'll go out on a limb and say that marijuana probably doesn't cause pathological penis shrinkage. But there are other risks that might be real. Lots of them.[20]

One is a so-called hyperemesis syndrome in which patients develop severe and persistent nausea, vomiting, and abdominal pain.[21] (That term comes from *emesis*, the Latin for vomiting.) The cause isn't known, and indeed this syndrome is a bit of a mystery because it *is* known that cannabinoids are effective in reducing nausea. The good news, though, is that the nausea seems to resolve when marijuana is stopped. Also, for unknown reasons, many people report relief from a hot bath or shower.

Moving on down the list of other risks we come to allergies. Everyone is allergic to something, and marijuana—particularly when it's smoked—has plenty of stuff in it that could cause an allergic reaction. Especially all of the stuff that goes up in smoke, like tar and bits of burnt plant matter.

Another possible risk is complications of pregnancy, especially since there's at least a theoretical reason to worry about these risks. For instance, we know that THC increases levels of a hormone called pregnenolone, which is a precursor of estrogen and other hormones.[22] Interestingly, pregnenolone also inhibits the CB1 receptor in a negative feedback loop.

But does that effect on hormones lead to pregnancy problems? The results here are conflicting. On one hand, there appears to be an increased risk of stillbirth among recreational marijuana users.[23] That effect is probably independent of other risk factors like cigarette smoking and alcohol use. However, those marijuana users may have been exposed to other drugs—or other risk factors—that were unknown. So it's not certain that marijuana is to blame.

Other studies make it even more difficult to draw any firm conclusions about marijuana use and pregnancy. For instance, one study found that marijuana use wasn't associated with pregnancy problems.[24] Although that's reassuring, another study found that marijuana use was associated with an increased risk of preterm birth, but only in women who were also smokers.[25]

Given these conflicting studies, it's impossible for me to figure out what marijuana's real pregnancy-related risks might be. That's especially true because all of the studies I've mentioned looked at recreational use of marijuana, not medical use. It's possible that those women used other illegal drugs, too, and that some of the risks these studies reported are due to those drugs. If that's true, then the real risks of marijuana are probably lower.

However, it's important to remember that people who are using marijuana for medical reasons might be using other (legal) drugs. Those drugs might carry pregnancy risks, too. And—what is particularly concerning—there might be interactions between those drugs and marijuana that we haven't discovered yet. So even though the evidence is mixed, there's probably enough reason to think twice about using marijuana during pregnancy.

The possibility of drug interactions isn't just limited to women who are pregnant. Think about all of the other drugs that people take every day. With THC and CBD and their metabolites, that's thousands of possible combinations. And somewhere in those pairings, there are probably some potential adverse reactions. But what kinds of reactions? We don't really know yet, but there are two big categories of interactions to watch out for.

The first is rather obvious. THC in particular can make you sleepy, so it's wise to avoid other drugs, such as high doses of opioids, or benzodiazepines, that also make you sleepy. Similarly, mixing alcohol and marijuana isn't a good idea. And, as we've seen, since marijuana can increase heart rate, it's probably wise to avoid other drugs that also increase heart rate, such as theophylline, or amphetamines (which are sometimes used to treat depression in patients with serious illness).

The second group of interactions is less obvious, but possibly more important. Many drugs are metabolized in the liver by enzymes in the cytochrome p450 family. These enzymes typically break a drug down into an inactive form, or one that is less active. And the key thing to know is that cannabinoids may inhibit that enzyme. So in theory, marijuana could increase the effective doses of many drugs, because they're not getting metabolized as quickly as they normally would.

Unfortunately, we don't know which drugs might be affected most. And we probably won't know until a lot more research is done. But perhaps the best advice is to assume that marijuana could alter the effects of other drugs, and to be alert for side effects.

Are there other risks of marijuana? Almost certainly. It's just difficult to sort through all of the reports to figure out what's real.

That's partly because the list of potential risks is astonishingly long. Some risks, such as decreased sperm count, are modest. Others are more significant, such as relatively benign heart rhythm problems like paroxysmal atrial fibrillation[26] and much more serious fatal arrhythmias.[27] There are also reports of blood vessel inflammation,[28] as well as inflammation of the heart muscle.[29]

Other reports have highlighted rare events. These include one-sided blindness due to a blockage in the eye's central retinal vein,[30] and fungal lung and brain abscesses.[31] Reports have also described unexplained stroke in young adults, and heartbeat pauses lasting almost six seconds.[32]

There have been reports, too, of slowed fetal growth in the second trimester.[33] In men, marijuana use might produce decreased testosterone levels,[34] and gynecomastia, a painful enlargement of breast tissue.[35] Pancreatitis has been reported,[36] as well as recurrent herpes infections, perhaps due to immune suppression.[37]

That's an exhaustive—and exhausting—list of risks. Some are probably real, and others aren't. Unfortunately, we just don't know enough right now to be able to figure out which ones we need to worry about.

So my best advice for most of these risks is to be wary. Listen carefully to reports of risks, especially if they come from large, controlled studies. But don't be paranoid, and keep an open mind.

Deconstructing a Gummy Bear

Most of the risks I've shown you are unavoidable. They're unavoidable, that is, unless you abstain from marijuana entirely. Indeed, the best way to make sure you don't have a marijuana-induced stroke or heart attack is to stay away from the stuff.

But there are two types of risks that we can avoid while still using marijuana. For instance, there's the risk of an unexpectedly high THC concentration, like what was in the joint that caused me to hear air traffic controllers in my living room. And there's a chance of contaminants, such as the insect legs that Steve was worried about.

These risks are real, but you can reduce them significantly, or avoid them entirely if you use marijuana that's been tested. Simple chemical analysis can tell you how much THC is in that piece of chocolate, or whether your joint has been contaminated by cricket feet. To see how chemical analysis works, I pay a visit to Cannlabs, a laboratory in Colorado that's made a highly successful business out of testing marijuana and marijuana-related products.

Cannlabs can tell you exactly what's in a joint or a bar of chocolate. They could have told me how much THC was in that joint I tried, and, presumably, they could have warned me that air traffic controllers in my living room were a potential risk.

On the second floor of a low, nondescript office building, Cannlabs' glass door reveals a neat office space with pristine carpeting and new furniture. I'm greeted by Heather Despres, the lab manager. Her blond hair is still damp from a morning shower, and delicate, rectangular glasses frame an open and friendly face. She's informally dressed in jeans and a ruffled blouse, with the wholesome aura of a manager of an organic marijuana dispensary. And that, as it turns out, is what she had always wanted to be.

Several years ago, Heather and a friend thought seriously about starting a marijuana dispensary, but the costs were prohibitive. And, she says, the business back then was like the Wild West. There was no quality control or assurances that patients were getting what they were promised. She tried a series of other jobs that made use of her skills as an analytic chemist until finally she discovered the growing business of marijuana testing.

"Now I finally feel like I'm in the right place. I'm doing a job that's important—we protect patients. And I'm using my skills to make the world a better place. How great is that?"

People bring in all sorts of things to be tested. There's the obvious, like buds, hashish, hash oil, wax, shatter, dab, lotions, patches, and tinctures. And there are also a lot of edibles—cookies, brownies, cake, crackers, hard candy, soda, taffy, potato chips, even milk shakes.

Testing everything is important, Heather says, because of safety and quality concerns, but also because you often don't know what you're going to get.

I tell her my back pain story, and she nods.

"Sure. Now that cannabis is getting more popular, and more common, more people are using it. People try it for the first time and they get a big surprise. You know what I mean?"

I do. My own experience with marijuana for medical purposes is an excellent argument for testing, which would have warned me that what I was about to smoke was industrial strength. And most medical marijuana consumers don't get much more information than I had. Some dispensaries test their products, but most don't.

That lack of testing, plus marijuana's increasing popularity, are probably responsible for a 30 percent increase in calls to poison control centers about marijuana toxicity from 2009 to 2010.[38] Interestingly, and more worrying, there was a similar increase in questions about marijuana exposures that involved kids under the age of thirteen.

The key, Heather tells me, is the dose. "Especially with THC, you have to know exactly what you're getting."

This is what I was curious about. How do you know how much THC is in a chocolate bar? Or in a joint delivered to your door by a lawyer friend of a friend, just for example. Can they test for THC?

"Sure. And other cannabinoids, too. CBD, obviously." Actually, they test for several. But most people are interested in THC and CBD, and their ratio.

"That's our job—we want to give people the information that they need to make the best possible decisions."

She explains that those decisions require information about dose, and also about safety. I'm curious about what "safety" means, aside from the obvious risk of an overdose.

"Oh boy," she says. "You don't want to know what might be in a product." She pauses. "Actually, you really do want to know. That's the point."

Such as?

"Well, you have your microbials. Like *E. coli*. And *Aspergillus*. And *Mucor* species."

E. coli is a common bacteria that's found in feces. But in tiny doses, it doesn't usually cause illness. *Aspergillus* is a fungus that's ubiquitous, but also doesn't usually result in illness. *Mucor* is a particularly bad actor, and systemic infections cause skin necrosis and terrible ulcers. However, even though *Mucor* is common in the environment, it doesn't usually cause illness, either.

These microbes are usually pretty harmless, so I'm not sure why she's so worried about them.

"Think about the patients who are using these products," she says. "They're sick. Some of them are very sick. They have compromised immune systems. Even small amounts of those sorts of contaminants can be fatal."

She's right. Patients with compromised immune systems as a result of chemotherapy or HIV, for instance, can't handle some microbes that would barely be noticeable in someone who is healthy. They also get illnesses from bacteria and fungus that don't cause problems in people whose immune systems are functioning normally. In fact, when certain organisms like *Listeria* or *Aspergillus* cause an infection, we usually search for an underlying immune problem. So microbial testing seems important, at least if you have a serious illness.

But what else do they test for?

"Well, it depends on what the product is. For flowers—cannabis— we test for pesticides."

Pesticides? I'm pretty sure that the expression on my face is a better argument for testing than anything the Cannlabs marketing team has created.

"Sure. Anything you use on a crop can come out in the finished product. Including," she adds, "a lot of chemicals you don't want to be inhaling."

There are lots of pesticides that might appear in marijuana, including organophosphates, organochlorides, and carbamates. Their effects on health are diverse and often controversial, but pesticide exposure in the short term has been associated with nausea, headaches, dizziness, and lung inflammation. Long-term effects include cancer, birth defects, and nerve damage.

And what else do they test for?

"Well, for the oils and concentrates, we look for solvents."

That's a relief. Some budder manufacturers, like Justin, use carbon dioxide. But others use naphthalene or butane or heptane. And Heather is saying that you really don't want any of those chemicals left in whatever you're smoking. Even in small amounts, many of those solvents are associated with an increased risk of cancer, and short-term exposure is associated with lung inflammation, nausea, headaches, and confusion.

Anything else?

There are a few other things they test for. Like aflatoxins. These are naturally occurring toxins that are produced by fungi like *Aspergillus*. They're present in trace amounts in groundnuts (like peanuts) and grains. Rarely, under the wrong conditions, there are enough of them to cause liver failure and death. Over the long term, they're also potent carcinogens that can cause liver cancer.

And particulates show up, too. Even something as seemingly benign as talc can be dangerous if it's burned and inhaled. The result can be lung damage that looks like an acute form of what miners get after years of exposure to coal dust.[39]

Do they find much?

"We find a lot," Heather says. "Way too much."

Marijuana Porn

We head down two flights of steps to the basement, through a freshly renovated waiting area with new furniture and wood flooring. It seems a little like a stage set that's been dropped into this old building. Heather punches a security code into a keypad and ushers me into her lab.

The walls are a bright, blinding white. The poured epoxy floor is squeaky clean, and two lab benches are scattered with shiny new machinery. It looks like a hospital testing lab.

Heather grins when I tell her this. That's what she wants to hear.

Immediately inside the door, there's a large wire rack that's packed with all sorts of samples. There are dozens of foil pouches. And a bewildering variety of boxes and packages and objects wrapped in plastic.

Heather explains that by law, samples need to be couriered. You can't send marijuana through the U.S. Postal Service, so all samples need to be dropped off. She also describes a chain of custody whose rigor seems to rival the process that's used for criminal evidence. Because of the costs of a courier service, many Cannlabs clients are dispensaries or growers or manufacturers, for whom testing is a business expense. But they also do testing for individuals. (Cal and Cindy told me they sent their CBD oil to Cannlabs to have it tested for CBD and THC concentrations before they gave it to their daughter Randi.)

On one bench there's an oversized monitor that's scrolling through images of, well, pretty much everything. There's a syringe filled with marijuana-infused oil. Then a cookie. And something that is clearly a bud. Then something else that looks like . . .

. . . a gummy bear?

Heather nods. "Like I told you, we get pretty much everything." She explains that these images on the large monitor are the pictures that another employee takes of the samples that come in.

A close-up of a bud flashes on the screen and Heather points. "He does great work. People like to call it marijuana porn."

After a sample sits for its portrait, it's registered and given a bar code. Then it's dissolved in solvent and sonicated, or subjected to high-frequency waves that break up solid substances such as gummy bears.

At this point things get technical. They use cultures and DNA assays for look for microbials, she says. And they use liquid chromatography to look for cannabinoids and other chemicals.

It's becoming obvious in our conversation that Heather would like to make testing mandatory for all marijuana products in all states in which it's legal. (At this time, for most states it's optional.) That makes me wonder—it's one thing to advocate for testing, but what happens if different labs test in different ways, say, with gas versus liquid chromatography, that produce different results?

"That's a problem," she admits. The laws in Colorado and indeed in many states don't standardize methods. Heather frowns, annoyed by this lack of consistency. For an analytic chemist who strives for order and regularity, this is making her unhappy.

"It's really a problem if a marijuana grower comes to us and says, 'Well, you told me my THC is 5 percent but I sent a sample to another lab and they're telling me it's 9 percent. Why should I believe *you*?'"

That's also a big problem when she tests for microbials.

"You get some people who say, 'I have the best stuff. The cleanest grow.'" She pauses. "Then they come up dirty. They're like, 'How is that possible?'"

From there, she says, reactions can go one of two ways. Some are in denial, and a few of them look for another lab. But others, Heather tells me, ask for help. Those customers are her favorite. "Maybe a grower comes up hot for *E. coli*," she says happily. "Where did that come from? Well, mostly from compost tea. A lot of the growers around here, they want to be all natural. All organic. No pesticides. But they make compost tea that uses all-natural ingredients, like earthworm castings."

(In case you're wondering, as I was, what earthworm castings are, they are feces. That is, earthworm droppings.)

Ick factor aside, the worm casings aren't what's producing the *E. coli*, Heather explains. It's the cow manure that growers blend with the casings to make a rich liquid—compost tea—that they spray all over the plants. The growers don't realize they're spraying their plants with *E. coli*.

Cannlabs recommends root drenching as an alternative to spray. Heather's particularly adamant about airflow. "Some places, they spray the compost tea all over the plants in an enclosed room and that room vents to the packaging area. So you're fumigating your clean packaging room with airborne *E. coli* and anything else." She makes a face that shows she strongly disapproves of this lapse in industrial hygiene.

Our tour draws to an end as Heather walks me out past the rack of incoming samples. There's just one more question I need to ask. I've been avoiding this one, but here goes.

At the end of the day, Cannlabs is left with all kinds of stuff, right?

The actual testing doesn't require a large sample. Often just a few grams. So if a dispensary submits a bag of gummy bears or a tray of brownies or an entire bud, where does the rest of it go?

I try to pose this question as delicately as I can, because it occurs to me that Heather might think I'm foraging for remnants. Indeed, she seems to scrutinize me a little more closely. But after a moment she relents. They have a flammable waste disposal contract, she explains. All waste is collected by a company that's then responsible for incinerating it.

So there you have it. At the end of the day, all of these joints and buds and brownies and gummy bears go up in smoke.

Bodily Harm?

Considering the risks of marijuana use I've laid out in this chapter, you could be excused for having either of two entirely opposite reactions. First, you could conclude that marijuana is dangerous and best avoided entirely, no matter what the use, recreational or medical. That would be an entirely natural response.

But you could also say that these are little more than isolated reports and theoretical risks. Heart attacks and infertility and pancreatitis and pesticides, and so on. They sound so dire as to be almost implausible. It might even occur to you, as it does to me, that if these risks were real, my entire college class should be dead by now. So you might ignore these risks entirely.

That's especially tempting because the risks in this chapter are mostly unrelated to the mind, and the way that our brain works. Unlike the psychological risks posed by marijuana use, like psychosis and addiction, these are physical risks. And while it's easy to imagine that marijuana could result in psychosis, it's not intuitively obvious that marijuana could result in pancreatitis or lung cancer.

It's tempting to choose one of these all-or-nothing reactions, either rejecting marijuana entirely or ignoring these risks. Indeed, many people weighing in about the legalization of medical marijuana tend to take one of these extreme positions. But that's not helpful. If you're trying to decide whether medical marijuana might be right for you, you probably want to know how it could help you, and how it might hurt you, so that you can make up your own mind.

Somewhere in the lists of risks I've described in this chapter, there will probably be some that turn out to be real. There probably won't be as many as marijuana's critics claim there are. But there will almost certainly be more than its most enthusiastic proponents admit.

Which ones? It's too soon for a final verdict, and it's almost impossible to know how we might avoid most of them. But I can offer a couple of recommendations.

First, the risks of contamination that Heather warned about are real. But that's not an indictment of medical marijuana. You could raise the same concerns about ground beef or packaged spinach. If anything, the risks of *E. coli* and pesticides are just a strong argument for mandatory testing and quality control. So let's put those aside and hope that there are lots of labs out there with chemists who are as compulsive as Heather is.

Second, there are other risks that we can't test our way around, including (reportedly) an increased risk of stillbirth or heart attack or stroke. We don't know for certain that these risks are real, but they're severe enough that we should take that possibility seriously.

But these, too, seem pretty manageable to me. Perhaps that's because I'm a hospice doctor and I'm used to prescribing drugs like morphine that have the potential for adverse effects and overdoses. And honestly, as I've pointed out, even drugs that are available over the counter have their risks.

For instance, diphenhydramine, an antihistamine, can cause dry mouth, blurred vision, sleepiness, constipation, and can make it difficult to urinate. It's also a common cause of severe confusion (delirium) in older adults. Those risks are significant, and yet diphenhydramine is sold over the counter, often under the brand name Benadryl, in the cold and allergy section of your local drugstore.

We can manage the risks of marijuana, just as we do the risks of other drugs. Some can be minimized by choosing patients carefully.

For instance, although I'd be the first to admit that the evidence about marijuana and pregnancy problems isn't entirely convincing, I wouldn't knowingly recommend marijuana to a woman who is pregnant. And patients who have other risk factors like high blood pressure or diabetes should at least be warned about other bad outcomes, such as heart attacks and strokes.

These recommendations may not be satisfying if you're looking for a clear and unambiguous verdict that marijuana is totally safe. Similarly, these recommendations probably aren't what you're looking for if you were hoping the evidence would prove once and for all that marijuana is a dangerous drug. The truth is somewhere in between.

That will change, though. And it will change in the next few years. In fact, I think it's safe to say that we're going to learn more—and more quickly—about medical marijuana's risks than we will about its benefits.

I said earlier that most of what we know about marijuana's risks comes from recreational users, and that's true. But as more people begin using marijuana for medical reasons, we'll be able to study their experiences, too. We'll learn about its short-term effects and long-term impact. Just as we know a lot about the risks of alcohol and tobacco, we'll come to understand the risks of marijuana much better than we do now.

8

Caveat Emptor

I've discovered that the science of medical marijuana is surprisingly complicated. For instance, there are a lot of different ways by which its active ingredients can be administered or ingested. And, as we've seen, some of those methods are more effective than others. How do patients figure out whether a joint is right for them? Or brownies? Or a vaporizer? And how do they figure out how much marijuana to use, and how often?

Then there are the benefits of marijuana. It seems to work well for some problems, like neuropathic pain, but less well for others. How do patients figure out whether marijuana could help them?

And of course there are risks of side effects, drug interactions, and adverse medical effects. Sorting through those risks was a challenge even for me, and I had the time and training to read studies critically. But most people don't have extensive medical training, so they're going to need help in figuring out what they should be concerned about and, possibly, how worried they need to be.

How are patients supposed to sort through all of this information to figure out whether marijuana could help them or hurt them? Can they expect helpful advice and guidance, or should the buyer beware (caveat emptor)?

When I started this book, I figured that even if marijuana wasn't helpful, at least it wasn't harmful. But I've changed my mind, and now I'm convinced both that there are risks and that there are real benefits. So it's important that all of the people who are turning to medical marijuana for help are getting good advice. But are they?

To find out, I decide to spend some time as a patient.

The Pot Doctor Will See You Now

I'm strolling down a sleepy, sun-drenched street in Southern California, past a used bookstore, a falafel restaurant, and a home brew supply store. Across the street there's a thrift shop, a pet store, and a jeweler. What I don't see, though, is the medical marijuana clinic I'm looking for.

Specifically, I'm looking for a medical marijuana clinic where I can obtain a letter of recommendation that will let me buy marijuana for medicinal purposes. And, if I'm lucky enough to score that letter, I want to know whether the doctor will offer me any advice that will help me figure out what to do with it.

I'm not actually planning to make a purchase. Let's be clear about that. (And to all of you DEA agents reading this, let me take this opportunity to say how much I appreciate all of the work that you do. Great job!)

But the best way for me to find out what patients are being told is for me to become a patient. At least for an hour.

I walk by the same nondescript storefront twice before I check the address and realize that this is the place I've been looking for. This "clinic" is noticeable mostly for its anonymity. This storefront is marked only by a plastic sign that's tethered to the building's façade. The sign is professionally done, but it also looks as though it could be taken down in a matter of minutes. This ability to close up shop in a hurry, I'm about to learn, might come in handy.

Inside there's a barren, linoleum-tiled space inhabited by a loose collection of plastic chairs pushed up against the left and right walls. Sitting on those chairs are five people who are about as different as people can possibly be. They're all facing each other, but studiously avoiding eye contact.

On my right, there's a beefy guy in his sixties with a goatee who is wearing a Harley T-shirt and worn denim overalls. Next to him are two waifish kids who might be Latino and who can't be much more than eighteen, wearing identical black zip-front hoodies. On my left, there's a tall, graying African American man in his forties who is bundled up in several layers of sweaters despite the near-tropical California weather outside and the lack of air-conditioning in here. Next to him is a pretty woman in her twenties reading a paperback copy of *The Grapes of Wrath*. She's the only one with any reading material. The others seem content to scrounge what diversion they can find in the patterns of the ceiling tiles overhead, which, for the record, are not that interesting.

Based on what we know about who uses medical marijuana, this cross section of humanity seems more diverse than what I expected. The largest study I've seen of patient characteristics was done right here in California.[1] Those researchers found that, compared to the general California population, medical marijuana patients were younger, more likely to be white, and had a higher level of education compared to the population as a whole. As I look around the waiting room I note that although this sample skews young and male, it is nevertheless quite diverse.

However, one group that does not seem to be represented in our little sample is a receptionist. Or a doctor. Or any authority figure.

"Just have a seat, man," the goateed guy says. "She'll come back when she comes back."

Before I can heed his counsel, a young blond woman emerges from the door behind the desk. She seems energetic and purposeful, but slightly flustered, too.

I'm a walk-in, I tell her.

She looks at me, one pierced eyebrow a quarter of an inch higher than the other, as if to say, "I can see that."

I tell her that I'd like to be evaluated for a letter of recommendation.

Now she's nodding, but still a little uncertainly. I'm suspecting that's because, honestly, why else would I be here? It's not the kind of place you'd come to have your cholesterol checked.

I wait five seconds, then ten. She's still thinking. Then—at last—she hands me a form on a clipboard and gestures toward a chair.

I sit down next to the pretty woman and look over the form. Among the initial questions is a space for either a social security number or a driver's license number. I'm thinking it would be unwise to share my social security number with this outfit, but divulging the latter will out me as a nonresident immediately. That, I know, will make me ineligible to get a letter of recommendation in California.

I can't believe they'll let me leave it blank. But, on the other hand, the pierced receptionist didn't ask me about my California residence. Nor did she ask to see my driver's license. So I turn to the second page.

This is where things get interesting. At the top, there's a big open space with a single, grammatically challenged question: "What symptoms for are you seeking relief?" (I'm learning that this is an industry in serious need of copyediting.)

What are my "symptoms for"? I'm thinking back to the study of California patients I mentioned earlier. In that group, pain was by far the most common reason for seeking medical marijuana. I figure my best strategy is to blend in, so I write "pain."

Then, in a flight of creativity I hope I won't regret later, I embellish with "low back pain." Just to make doubly sure, I add "chronic," underlined twice.

But this clinic obviously doesn't trust patients to generate their own symptoms. Further down the page, it offers suggestions, helpfully presented as check boxes. For instance, there's a list of past injuries that includes motorcycle accidents, bicycle accidents, car accidents, and "other."

I check them all.

I turn the page, and there are more. Lots more. This is going to be easy.

Back pain, ear problems, insomnia, headaches. I think I could come up with at least a partial justification for all of these. Check.

I pause on one: "Disturbing feelings." I'm not sure what that means, but find I'm disturbed by that ambiguity. Check.

Finally, again, there's "Other." Oddly, this option doesn't offer a space to write in the symptom that's bothering you. It's just a lone check box. So I check it.

As I turn in the clipboard to the receptionist, I take the opportunity to ask a practical question. If I don't qualify, is there a reduced fee?

She looks surprised for a moment. "If you don't qualify?" she asks. "Well, if that was to happen, then no, I guess we wouldn't charge you anything." She's still smiling in a perplexed way, as if failure to qualify is an outcome with which she is wholly unfamiliar.

Then she glances at my form. Her eyes scan the missing social security/driver's license information. She picks up a pen and fills in what appear to be random numbers. It's at this point that I begin to suspect that I'm in.

I sit back down and wait. Every five or ten minutes the receptionist calls out a name and sends one of my fellow supplicants through the door behind her. They go in, but they don't come out. First, the goateed man disappears. Then the guy in the sweaters. Then the young Latino guys in hoodies, together. I find this disappearance without reappearance is enhancing my disturbing feelings. I make a note to mention this to the doctor, if I ever meet him or her.

At least I have something to pass the time. I'm reading the text of California's Compassionate Use Act to find out which conditions it covers. Actually, what I really want to know is what's *not* covered, because the list of conditions is rather long, and bewilderingly open-ended.

The goal of the Compassionate Use Act, it promises, is "to ensure that seriously ill Californians have the right to obtain and use marijuana for medical purposes where the medical use is deemed appropriate and has been recommended by a physician."

The act lists cancer, anorexia, AIDS, and chronic pain. It also mentions spasticity, glaucoma, arthritis, and migraine. What is most helpful, though, is its allusion to "any other illness for which marijuana provides relief."[2]

Wondering what an "other illness" might be? Well, as we've seen, marijuana seems to be effective for a few conditions like neuropathic pain and nausea and perhaps others. But doctors' websites are much more creative in offering suggestions. I printed out several lists as I was searching the Internet last night. Premenstrual syndrome, for instance, was mentioned often. Diabetes and asthma showed up on most doctors' lists. So did the all-inclusive "sports injury." Sample a random guy out on the street, and you're bound to find that he's got at least one of these.

That's an almost all-inclusive list. And as we've seen, there haven't been many clinical trials of marijuana. So I can't believe that each of these symptoms is a legitimate indication for a recommendation. But presumably I can ask the doctor. If I ever meet him.

Finally, the pierced receptionist calls my name. Somewhat unnecessarily, since we're the only two people in the room. But I have to respect her commitment to protocol.

I stand. She beckons. I follow her through the door of promise.

Once I'm through that door, though, I'm disappointed to find that the inner sanctum is nothing but a small windowless cube with fake wood paneling and an exceptionally low particleboard ceiling hovering just above our heads. The combined effect of the close walls and low ceiling gives the illusion of stepping into some Alice in Wonderland universe that is about half the size of the regular one.

In the center of the room is a battered particleboard desk that looks like it was birthed by a chance coupling between an IKEA table and a box of Lincoln Logs. Behind it is a thin, gray-bearded man with flyaway hair in a dirty white coat.

I smile, but he doesn't look up. Then the receptionist disappears to guard the waiting room and I take a closer look at the doctor as I settle into a metal folding chair. He must be at least ninety years old. Personal hygiene doesn't seem high on his daily priority list. His rumpled white coat has brown stains at the cuffs and collar, and he's wearing a frayed open-neck plaid shirt with enormous collar wings that seem to engulf his scrawny neck. He also has a pen behind each ear. And he's holding a third.

The doctor still hasn't introduced himself. Nor has he looked up at me. Instead, he's busily reviewing my application, peering out from under unkempt-hedgerow eyebrows. He seems to be circling every symptom and diagnosis that I've checked. So far, so good.

Then the doctor starts asking me rapid-fire questions that are initially confirmatory. Headaches? Back pain? He's going so fast I only have time to nod.

Then he switches to questions that come in seemingly random clusters of three symptoms. He's like a one-armed-bandit slot machine channeling a medical dictionary:

"Constipation, headaches, nausea?"

"Cancer, weight loss, fever?"

"Palpitations, diarrhea, joint pain, anything like that?"

I'm having trouble thinking of a category of conditions that encompasses palpitations, diarrhea, and joint pain. So I just shake my head.

Undeterred, he adds a few more circles to my application and nods, satisfied. Then he turns to the last page of my application and scribbles an illegible signature at the bottom. The receptionist has already filled in my name, so the sheet of paper that the doctor pushes across the desk is complete.

This approval, the letter says, is for "a significant medical condition." I'm still not sure what that condition is.

I ask the doctor whether he thinks that marijuana might help me.

"Might," he says. And he shrugs.

For pain?

"Might," he says again. Then: "Might not."

The doctor takes the pen from behind his left ear and places it on the form. Then he pushes himself up using the arms of his chair, and picks up a cane that had been leaning against the other side of the desk. With a clumsy grace, he hobbles over to the door and knocks. Then he's back in his chair sitting across from me.

He points to the recommendation. Indeed, there's a place for my signature at the bottom of the page, where I attest that I have been warned, among other things, that "marijuana is a medicine, for appropriate use only."

And there's another warning: "When using medical cannabis, I will not drive or operate heavy machinery." All right, I think I can agree to that. I sign.

Apparently we're done. I stand up just as the receptionist comes in. Somehow, she managed to leave through the back door and come back in through the front.

"I'll take you to our dispensary." She gestures toward the back door.

Ah. Now the strange disappearances make sense. The receptionist has been walking the other patients to the clinic's dispensary so they can pay. And, presumably, so they can make a purchase.

I find out later that this is a common business strategy. The "consultation" I just went through was a loss leader that got me in the door. The real money gets made at the next step, with the actual purchase. The receptionist, still holding my form, ushers me out the back door and into blinding sunlight.

The dispensary proves to be as seedy as the clinic I've just visited. Samples appear in battered glass cases, incense smolders in a corner, and Bob Marley plays at earsplitting volume. So I pay my thirty-dollar fee and beat a hasty retreat.

I can't say with certainty that this is typical of what patients experience when they get a recommendation for medical marijuana. In fact, I hope it isn't. But from what I've heard, it's not that unusual. Many of the patients I've met describe similar encounters. For instance, there's often not a lot of diagnosing going on. And advice is rare, beyond the simple recommendation to use marijuana.

I'll go out on a limb and guess that the vast majority of patients will find it as easy as I did to get a recommendation, if they're in a state in which it's legal. But they won't get any help figuring out whether and how marijuana might help them. So in many states, medical marijuana is still very much a do-it-yourself proposition.

The Woman Who Wanted to Be in Control

Surely there are clinics trying to provide useful advice, or dispensaries that function like pharmacies, at which you can both buy marijuana products and learn how to use them. Indeed there are. It takes me a while, but eventually I meet Lisa, who tells me about a clinic, and a dispensary, which changed her life.

The first thing I notice about Lisa is how fragile she seems. Her narrow face, pale blue eyes, and thinning blond hair make her seem worn and weathered. If you met her on the street you'd guess that she has a serious illness. But you'd be surprised, as I was, to learn that she's only in her twenties.

Lisa has systemic lupus erythematosis, an autoimmune disorder that causes arthritis, fatigue, fevers, and which can lead to lung and kidney damage. I met her through a friend who told me that I really needed to hear Lisa's story about marijuana. I'm curious about that story, and about how she thinks marijuana helps her.

"I can't live without it," Lisa tells me. Actually, she says this several times in our conversation, in slightly different ways. It really helps her anxiety, she tells me. And when she's less anxious, the pain in her joints is more tolerable because she's not so tense. It's helped her so much, in fact, that now she takes Percocet only once a week, when she really needs it, whereas two years ago she was taking it around the clock.

What's striking about Lisa's story is that she tells me she uses medical marijuana because it gives her control. She can decide whether to use it, and when to use it, and how much she needs. She doesn't have to rely on a doctor, or anyone else.

"I'm in charge," Lisa says.

She goes on to tell me about the challenges she faced in visits to doctor after doctor, who didn't seem willing—or able—to help her find relief for her symptoms. Then she found what she describes as "the best clinic in the world." And the best dispensary. They put her back in charge of her health.

What are these places? They sound magical. And much different than what I experienced in that storefront clinic.

"I'll introduce you."

Sasha the Wonder Dog

After a brief nap, Sasha the Wonder Dog is back on patrol. She'd been taking a nap, but now she's at work, pacing the small waiting room of the United Health and Wellness clinic as if she owns the place. She pretty much does.

Sasha is an imposing shepherd mix with long, caramel-colored fur and the sweet disposition of a basset hound. She's also endowed with enormous ears the size and shape of twin radar dishes. They swivel in unison when anything catches her attention.

Those ears are swiveling now, and their activity is explained a few moments later when Larry Gidaley, her owner and the clinic's manager, steps through the door bearing an extra-large pizza. Sasha goes through contortions of excitement, then seems to remember her place as the dignified face of the clinic and calms down. She shadows Larry to a back room.

This medical marijuana clinic is in a nondescript industrial park outside downtown San Diego. It's up a flight of stairs from an entrance that does little to advertise itself, which seems to be intentional. To get here, you need to find the clinic online and you have to do your homework. You can't just wander in off the street, the way I did at the last clinic I visited. And that's the way Gidaley wants it.

The clinic itself is unpretentious. It's clean and well maintained, with a small waiting room that seats twelve. There's classic rock playing in the background at a modest level, fresh industrial carpet on the floor, recent magazines on the coffee table, and Saint Patrick's Day shamrocks everywhere.

To the right of the front door there's a sliding glass window that leads to the receptionist's space, and next to that is a cannabis resource center—a large rack of pamphlets and business cards for dispensaries. Unlike the other clinic I visited, Larry's doesn't sell marijuana or related products. Around the corner are three other offices, for storage, for the physician consultation, and for office staff. That's about it.

It turns out that Sasha is emblematic of the clinic's warm and friendly customer service that is more typical of a nice hotel than a medical clinic. For instance, Larry and his wife, Debbie, greet patients as they come in, offering ice water and a warm welcome. Larry also makes a point of asking if anyone has a problem with dogs, although it's difficult to imagine that anyone would have a problem with this one.

Then there are the baked goods. When I arrived earlier, Debbie greeted me with a hug and an offer of fresh blueberry muffins. Normally I'm not one to pass up baked goods, but Larry had informed me proudly that Debbie is a wizard at incorporating marijuana into culinary items, including his favorite, linguini with clam sauce. So I eyed that muffin with more than a little apprehension. (It was entirely safe.)

There's also a friendly camaraderie among the staff and patients. Larry, Debbie, and Kaylie the medical assistant show a real concern about patients' symptoms, for instance. And they offer friendly hugs of greeting for return customers, of which there are many. It feels a little like a cross between a clinic and a block party. In fact, it's exactly the sort of "relational" clinic experience that Steve Lankenau thinks might provide support and might even reduce the risk of addiction.

The result is that this waiting room crowd is more diverse than that of any other clinic I've visited. When I arrive, three chairs are filled by tough, lean guys with tattoos and jeans and work boots and suntans that looked like they've been burned in by years of outdoor work. Next to them are an elderly Chinese man and his grandson. And then a young woman and her five-year-old son.

And the level of naïveté here is astonishing. Conservatively, I'd say that half of the patients I meet are new to the world of medical cannabis. One overheard conversation between a carefully groomed woman in her fifties and Kaylie:

Kaylie: "These are the regulations for growing."

Woman: "Growing?"

Kaylie: "Marijuana."

Woman: "Oh!" Sharp intake of breath. "I didn't know you're allowed to grow marijuana. Well, I'll be darned."

That exchange says a lot about this clinic, maybe more than Larry's warm welcome, or Sasha's patrols, or even Lisa's recommendation. People who wouldn't set foot in the first clinic that I visited would feel comfortable here. For instance, Alice, the woman who used marijuana to get to sleep, got her recommendation here.

Patients at United Health and Wellness can expect advice that's both thorough and thoroughly nonmedical. That is, patients don't get a prolonged visit with a doctor and a physical examination. In fact, their only contact with a physician is a video consultation with a doctor in another state.

This is a common practice, and allows a single physician to see dozens of patients every day. So even at this clinic, which is among the nicest I've visited, patients don't get a lot of direct advice. They go through a checklist that's similar to the one that I filled out, albeit with much better grammar and punctuation. There are clinics that operate just as regular medical clinics do, with a half hour or more of face time with a physician, and even a physical exam. But the quick interview and checklist seems to be the most common model.

But what patients at this clinic don't get from a doctor, they can get from the staff, and from each other. Indeed, the friendly camaraderie of this place seems designed to encourage people to swap stories and share advice. I overhear conversations about the benefits of CBD oil for one woman's muscle spasms, for instance, and about how a new *indica* strain is the best for sleep. There's advice, too, about how to deal with mandatory drug testing at work, and about how to explain medical marijuana use to friends and family members. So even though the doctor provides little more than a slip of paper and a signature, patients like Lisa leave with more advice and support than most doctors could offer.

"The Drug That Big Pharma Doesn't Want You to Know About"

The United Health and Wellness clinic helped Lisa feel like she's in control, but she only goes to that clinic once a year to renew her recommendation. Instead, it's the marijuana dispensary that she really depends on for advice. So, on her next trip, she invites me along.

Now Lisa is leading me through a nondescript door and down a long, narrow hallway. There's light ahead, and I can hear the music of sitars and tambourines undulating in what sounds like an endless loop. Then we're in a bright, clean room.

Against one wall are flat glass-topped counters of the sort that you'd find in a jewelry store. Posters of cannabis plants line the walls, as do several anatomy posters, including one that displays the brain in excruciating detail.

There's also a large, bearded man waiting behind the counter. Lisa leans over the display case, immediately engrossed in reviewing its contents, which are just inches from her nose. The man introduces himself as Allen.

Lisa takes a step back and points to me. We haven't rehearsed this, but she knows I have my recommendation with me. And on the drive over she told me I should be a patient in order to get to see how wonderful this dispensary is.

"Be a patient. Just like me."

So I'm up. Of course, I'm not planning to make a purchase. I'm pretty sure I haven't broken any laws yet, since I was truthful with that sleazy clinic about both my symptoms and residency status. But I have no intention of using this fraudulently obtained piece of paper to buy anything.

Allen is looking at me expectantly, so I say I'm not quite ready to buy yet, which is technically true. He nods. Apparently window-shopping is common in this market. I say that I'm just trying to get a sense of what's available.

A mercenary salesperson would cut me loose and move on to the next customer, but Allen segues smoothly from salesman to teacher, and tells me he's been a user for more than twenty years. And his demeanor indicates that nothing would give him greater pleasure than to teach me about what he refers to several times as "the drug that Big Pharma doesn't want you to know about." Then he asks me my name with the frank, getting-to-know-your-client tone of a neighborly insurance agent.

"Well, Dave, let's take a look." And he glances over the recommendation form that I've handed him. He scans the list, nodding. Right now, I'm wishing fervently that I hadn't checked "disturbing feelings."

"So you're just starting out?" He doesn't wait for a reply. I think one look at me is enough to tell him that I'm not a user with a twenty-year history.

"For back pain and insomnia, I'd definitely go with an *indica* strain. Something mild at first." (The *indica* strains, remember, generally have less THC and more CBD, and therefore lack the hard-hitting psychoactive effects of *sativa* strains.)

He pulls five small plastic trays out of a case. Each is about four inches square and is piled with a generous sample, enough marijuana to get you a ten-year prison sentence in many jurisdictions. They're helpfully labeled with little tent signs.

I look more closely and am surprised by how different they are. For instance, the one on my far left is Holy Grail Kush. It's greenish brown with the texture of granola, and has walnut-sized nuggets spiked with tiny orange filaments that look like cotton candy. Right next to it is another pile labeled "Northern Lights." It's lighter, almost tan, with much smaller nuggets, about the size of popcorn. It also has what seems like a heavy layer of sugar frosting. (It's not just me. A quick consultation with Lisa confirms that these buds really do look like food.)

With the practiced eye of an experienced salesperson, Allen notes my interest in the left end of the row.

"Yeah, good call. The Holy Grail is a good starter bud. Mellow and slow. Not much of an active buzz. Very calming." He nudges it forward. "Take a sniff."

I sniff. It smells like . . . lemon?

Allen nods. "Lemon and citrus—you can smell it even at room temperature. It really comes through when you light up, though."

He pauses, looking down the rest of the lineup.

"That's probably your best option, to start. I mean, you could try the Northern Lights, I guess. It's 100 percent *indica*, and they've got the genetics to prove it. But it's weird—it smokes more like a hybrid."

He means that the grower has promised him that, genetically, this strain is 100 percent *Cannabis indica*, the species that is known for having a high concentration of CBD, without much THC. But it has some of the psychoactive effects of a *sativa* strain that emphasizes THC.

Just for completeness, Allen spins me through the other options on the table. "There's Chunkle," he says, pointing to the next in line. "Mild. Very mild. Great as a starter. But maybe too mild for you?"

I nod, trying to be helpful.

"Right. Then there's LA Confidential. Bit more of a head buzz than maybe you want the first time out. OK for insomnia, though, and really great for pain. Absolutely tops. That's why I've used it." Allen barely looks down at my application, which he seems to have memorized.

"Yeah," he says, "I had some tough back pain, too, a couple of years ago. Just moved in the wrong direction and I was laid out with the spasms. It was the worst pain I ever had. But I had some LA Confidential and I fired it up. It was a miracle."

He smiles at the memory. I'm thinking that's the only time I've ever heard a middle-aged man reminisce fondly over an episode of acute back pain, or at least the relief from it.

"And last," Allen says, "there's White Widow. Of course."

White Widow is the classic *indica* strain, said to be sedating to the point of immobilization. I've heard that the stronger varieties can put injudicious users into a state of near catatonia for eight hours or more. It's not for the unwary. Allen seems to subscribe to that opinion.

"It's a classic," he says simply. "But it'll knock you on your ass. Better save that for later."

I ask if any of them is safer than the others.

Allen laughs. "They're all safe, man. Cannabis is a flower. Not like narcotics."

Apparently Allen has forgotten that opiates—narcotics—are derived from poppies. And that poppies are, in fact, flowers.

Even though Allen is sanguine about the risks of this stuff, he's still suggesting I start slow. "For now I'd go with the Holy Grail. Or maybe the Chunkle, if you really want to start out slow. But honestly, I'd go with the Holy Grail to get some relief, then fill in with the Chunkle in between. You know, like use the Holy Grail when you really need it, after a long day or on weekends, and then hit the Chunkle in the morning, or while you're working."

I'm not sure what sort of work the average user does. However, I'm pretty sure what I do as a physician is not compatible with firing up a joint first thing in the morning—or at any time, for that matter.

Still, I'm impressed by his advice. And I'm really impressed by the time he took with me—a noncustomer. But I really want to see how he handles Lisa, a real patient.

The Marijuana Sommelier

Now Lisa and Allen are talking about specific strains of marijuana. Allen mentions White Widow to Lisa, too, and follows up with Master and White Rhino, making this sound less like a consultation and more like a brainstorming session for a new Joss Whedon movie.

I'm eavesdropping intently because I want to know what Lisa finds so helpful here. What I overhear is a complex discussion of "buzz characteristics."

Lisa says she's finding it very hard to relax at the end of the day. It's a combination, she says, of stress at work and the pain in her muscles and joints that never leave her alone. She wants relief, but doesn't want to get high. She says she's looking for something "clean" and "fresh."

"But not goofy?" Allen asks.

She shudders. "No, not so much medication effect at all. Calming and soothing." She pauses. "I guess I'm looking for more of a body high, with a strong couch lock."

"And you want something that will help you sleep, too?" Allen guesses.

"Yeah, exactly."

He nods knowingly. It's that last term—"couch lock"—that got his attention. Something clicks in his expert mind.

His confident nod reminds me of the way that a wine sommelier will smile when you say something like, "I'm looking for a white that's low in fruit with a good nose and a dry finish. Something like a Napa Chardonnay, but without all the oak."

"You want . . ." Allen reaches down into the case between them. "Tuna Kush." He nods. "It's a hybrid but it smokes like pure *indica*. Not much buzz, more of a creeping effect. But take it slowly, a little at a time." He nods again.

Their conversation goes on for another fifteen minutes as I listen. Allen and Lisa talk about other strains. But they keep coming back enthusiastically to the Tuna Kush, despite a name that sounds—to me at least—like some obscure Afghan brand of cat food.

They talk about delivery methods, too. Allen asks Lisa about how she uses her marijuana—a series of conversational questions about method (vaporizer), brand (Volcano), timing (generally in the evenings), and frequency (once or twice a day; more on weekends). Along the way, he gives her advice about vaporizing technique, how to clean her vaporizer, how to grind the marijuana she uses, and proper temperature settings.

They also discuss other forms of marijuana, including edibles. Again, Allen goes through a series of careful questions to elicit Lisa's preferences, including what she likes and doesn't like about her Volcano. Although Allen was initially enthusiastic about edibles for her, when he heard that she liked the immediate relief of a vaporizer, he recommended against them.

"So I really think the Tuna Kush is a good choice for you, and I'd stick with the vaporizer," he says finally.

Lisa nods, apparently convinced. And not just convinced, but satisfied. This is what she was looking for. Not just the recommendation, but also the conversation. Especially the questions.

Now as she walks out the door of this dispensary, Lisa is carrying a paper bag whose contents will let her take control of her own symptoms. Specifically, she'll be able to treat them according to her needs and preferences. And she's confident that she's doing everything she can to manage her symptoms. As she leaves, she tells me that finding this place has been one of the best things that's ever happened to her.

Caveat Emptor

Lisa's is a success story. She finally found something that could help her manage her symptoms. And she got back at least some of the sense of control that her illness had taken from her.

But Lisa was lucky. Because if she'd had to rely on the clinic that I went to on my own, she probably wouldn't have gotten any useful advice or support—or sense of control.

It's tempting to interpret her story as a gentle caution. Perhaps we need to make sure all medical marijuana clinics and dispensaries are staffed by competent, knowledgeable people with good interpersonal skills. And maybe they should all have Wonder Dogs, too.

That's a start, but it's not enough. The stakes are too high to let some clinics do what they want. As we've seen, the benefits of marijuana are not clear-cut, and prospective patients need guidance and advice in figuring out what will work for them. Moreover, the risks of marijuana are real, and many are scary. So prospective patients will need help to understand those risks and to figure out which are worth worrying about.

I didn't get any of that from the first clinic I visited. I received no advice, or instructions, except a routine warning not to drive or operate heavy machinery. All I got was a letter of recommendation that no one should have given me, an out-of-state resident.

So if medical marijuana is going to be widely legal—and it certainly looks as though that's the trend—then these clinics and dispensaries are going to have to do much better. They're profiting off the legalization of medical marijuana as an officially sanctioned "drug," which is fine. But clinics and dispensaries need to be held to the same standards of quality control and oversight and education to which we hold medical pharmacies and clinics. Medical marijuana is becoming too widespread, and the risks are too great, to leave the patient to fend for herself, and let the buyer beware.

9

The Future of Medical Marijuana

I've told you what we know about whether marijuana works and how it might help us. I've told you, too, about some of its potential risks.

But what about the future? What could marijuana do for us someday? What might this plant contribute to medicine?

That is arguably the most interesting question of this book. But it's also the most difficult to answer, because marijuana isn't a drug. At least, it's not a drug in the same way that morphine or penicillin are drugs.

I've been able to show you what THC and CBD do, but a typical joint has dozens of cannabinoids in it, each with slightly different effects. And of course, some of those molecules don't do anything. So in order to figure out what marijuana might do for us in the future, we need to understand how those molecules work.

This might also be the most far-reaching question in this book. Up until now, we've seen what marijuana can do. And we've seen some of the effects, good and bad, of marijuana's two main ingredients, THC and CBD.

But that's really just one small piece of how cannabinoids work. If we really want to understand what they can do for us, we need to understand how they interact with receptors in our brains and our bodies. This is the next step in the science of medical marijuana, and it's one that promises enormous benefits for many of the symptoms and problems we've explored.

Alas, taking that step requires an exploration of several of the subjects that we all probably slept through in school, or skipped entirely: organic chemistry, anatomy, and neurophysiology. But first, there will be chocolate, because that's where the future of marijuana begins.

Ms. Sweet and Her Psychoactive S'more

"Oh. My. God. Chocolate cupcakes will get you so . . . *high!*"

Indeed? I had no idea. So many topics are missing from the medical school curriculum. Although I spent weeks memorizing the names of the bones in the foot, I can't recall a single lecture devoted to the hallucinogenic properties of baked goods.

But it must be the truth; anyway, the young woman standing in front of me—we'll call her Ms. Sweet—seems convinced of it. She's wearing an expression of rapt worship as she extolls the euphoric benefits of cupcakes in particular and the common cocoa bean in general. So I'm inclined to believe her.

Or at least I might, if she weren't also wearing a pink T-shirt with glittery letters that read: KIND OF SWEET, KIND OF NUTTY. So I'll reserve judgment for now. But I'm intrigued.

Fortunately, Ms. Sweet's claim is testable. We're standing outside a storefront in Santa Monica whose sign is a white puffy cloud with scalloped edges. It looks a little like a cartoon depiction of heaven, and has an aura of the psychedelic sixties.

Apparently Ms. Sweet knows this store well, and she opens the door with an easy familiarity, beckoning me inside. The interior is bizarre, even by the rather loose standards of Southern California. For instance, the first features that greet us are foot-wide vertical blue and white stripes on the front of the counter facing the door, and a black-and-white checkerboard on the wall.

It looks a little like what you'd get, say, if M. C. Escher barfed.

Perhaps to reassure customers who step into this visually disorienting mess, the young woman behind the counter is assertively pleasant, energetic, and friendly. She has long brown hair and is quite beautiful in an earthy way. On a cord around her neck she's wearing a polished stone that's mesmerizing.

The pretty woman behind the counter is looking at me expectantly. But how to put this delicately? Do they use a secret ingredient?

She smiles thinly and shakes her head, looking a little offended. Her left hand reaches for the stone hanging around her neck and she rubs it nervously.

"It's all natural," she says primly. "Just organic, and pretty much everything we sell is raw and unprocessed."

OK, I get that. Organic, natural, raw, and unprocessed. But those adjectives could be applied to lots of substances, including marijuana. I'm sensing a potential loophole. Those brownies on the top shelf?

"Nope."

They're not . . .

"Sorry."

Not even a little?

"No."

These baked goods may not have any marijuana in them, but Ms. Sweet's faith in the buzzworthiness of cupcakes and S'mores is based on something else entirely. Specifically, her high hopes are based on a psychoactive substance that *is* plainly advertised: anandamide.

Because that's the odd name of this place. The store's name caught my attention because anandamide is a neurotransmitter. And it's unusual, in my experience, for a bakery to be named after a neurotransmitter. Even in Santa Monica.

Anandamide isn't just any neurotransmitter. It's one of a class of neurotransmitters known as endocannabinoids. These are naturally occurring molecules that are often described as the body's own versions of THC and CBD. There are other neurotransmitters in this group, most notably 2-Arachidonoylglycerol, known to its friends as 2-AG.

2-AG is more potent than anandamide, and present in the body in larger amounts, but anandamide was discovered first. And, frankly, it has a better name. Anandamide is derived from the Sanskrit word for bliss, *ananda*, so it's known as the "bliss molecule." Inevitably, it gets more attention.

Anandamide isn't just a neurotransmitter. It's also present in some foods, notably cacao beans, the principal ingredient of chocolate. In fact, it was first found in chocolate in 1996.[1]

For the sake of completeness, I should mention that the researchers who found anandamide in chocolate also found two other compounds, N-oleoylethanoloamine and N-linoleoylethanolamine. But they would make lousy names for a bakery.

Ms. Sweet's hopes of a buzz, however, are unrealistic. There's generally only about 10 micrograms of anandamide in a gram of chocolate. If anandamide is about as potent as THC is, I figure you'd need about two kilograms of chocolate (20 milligrams of anandamide) to have any effect. Even if anandamide is much more potent than THC, you'd still need a lot of chocolate.

I won't tell her that, though. She's oohing and aahing and taking deep sniffs, her nose buried in the paper bag. She rolls her eyes and smiles the happy smile of someone who is having a very good day.

"Oh. My. God. My fingers are tingling." Ms. Sweet takes a deep breath from the bag. Then another. "Don't you feel the buzz?"

Alas, I don't. I'm not sure she does, either. I think she's just hyperventilating.

The THC Inside All of Us

Anandamide isn't just a (theoretical) way to get high on brownies. It's the star of the body's endocannabinoid system. Even more important, anandamide is the key to understanding how the ingredients in marijuana do what they do, and what those ingredients might do for us in the future.

When you smoke marijuana, THC and CBD do their thing by mimicking anandamide and 2-AG. That is, they work in the same way that drugs like morphine work, by mimicking molecules that we all have. Our bodies weren't designed to respond to morphine per se. And our bodies don't have "morphine receptors." But our bodies *are* designed to respond to enkephalins, which are hormones that have a variety of effects, including pain relief.

So morphine and many other related drugs exert their effects on our brains by acting on these enkephalin receptors. In the same way, the cannabinoids in marijuana exert their effects by acting on receptors that are designed for anandamide and other endocannabinoids. That is, you could say that they work by hacking the endocannabinoid system that we're born with.

The anandamide molecule was discovered in 1992 by the Israeli scientist Raphael Mechoulam, whom I introduced you to earlier, along with his students and collaborators. Their discovery proved to be a key turning point in our understanding of how marijuana works.

To give you a little perspective, it helps to know that most neurotransmitters in the brain were discovered in the 1930s, 1940s, and 1950s. The first one, acetylcholine, was discovered even earlier, in the 1920s, by Otto Loewi. But researchers stumbled on the endocannabinoid system much later. In fact, it wasn't until the 1990s that Mechoulam and William Devane made the discovery that would change the way we think about marijuana and how it might help us.[2]

Mechoulam had been hunting for anandamide for a long time. He hadn't found it yet, but he kept looking. He persevered because he knew that it had to exist, for two reasons.

First, he'd already produced several synthetic cannabinoids. These are molecules that look a little like THC and CBD, but are manufactured in a test tube. (Nabilone, the nausea treatment, is one of the best-known examples.)

Mechoulam learned that in order for those synthetics to work in the brain, they needed to have an exact structure and size—generally with one or two carbon rings and a long carbon tail. That is, his synthetics only worked when they fit a preexisting pattern. So he suspected that our bodies had a selective receptor, and that it was designed to bind to a particular molecule.

That hunch turned out to be correct. As Mechoulam was puzzling over this problem, two researchers on his team, Allyn Howlett and William Devane, found a cannabinoid receptor in rat brains that would later prove to be the CB1 receptor that binds to THC. So Mechoulam figured that the cannabinoids in marijuana worked by binding to that receptor, and that the receptor was designed to bind to one and only one molecule.

There was a second reason Mechoulam was convinced that there was a "natural" THC molecule in the body, and that reason is not as obvious, but more important. He knew that cannabinoid receptors are conserved across species. For instance, rat and human receptors are almost identical. So Mechoulam deduced that if different species have the same structure for their receptors—that is, if these receptors are a "conserved trait"—only a few molecules bind to them.

Are you with me? No?

Think about it this way: It's your first visit to a city and you're trying to take the subway for the first time. But there's a problem. You can't figure out how to pay. The turnstiles have slots in them, but those slots are an odd size. They're too narrow for a credit card, and they're too thin for a coin. But—and this is the most important point—these slots are all identical.

Increasingly frustrated, you try another station, with the same result. And another. Everywhere there are the same oddly shaped slots.

Eventually, after the third failure, you conclude that this subway system uses some form of card. One card will get you into a subway station anywhere. All you need to do is figure out what that card is (and where to buy one). Then you're in business.

That was Mechoulam's problem. He knew there had to be a neurotransmitter that was conserved across species, in the same way that those identical slots seemed to accept the same mysterious subway card. But what could it be?

To figure that out, he hired William Devane, one of the researchers who identified the CB1 receptor. Together they embarked on what would become a major project to find endogenous compounds that would bind to that receptor.

As to exactly *how* they did it, I can give you the CliffsNotes version. Basically, the research team took pig brains. Then—and I'm using some creative license here—they threw them into a blender. Next, they took extracts of the resulting mulch and ran it through a gas chromatograph, which separates molecules by size. Finally, they took the resulting groups, or "fractions," and tested each of them to see which one would prevent a synthetic form of THC from binding to receptors. They reasoned that anything that would block the synthetic THC from binding to a receptor was probably also, itself, capable of binding to that receptor.

Success. They found a molecule that they thought was a pretty good fit, literally. They had a molecule that seemed to bind to receptors in much the same way that THC does. That molecule—the "natural" version of THC—was anandamide.

Of course, Mechoulam already knew about CB1 and CB2 receptors, but this discovery was much bigger. By finding the molecule that those receptors are meant to bind to, he and his team were able to begin to study the system of molecules and receptors in each of us that THC and CBD tap into.

Once the researchers knew that there were natural cannabinoids in pigs, and people, they started looking in other species, and they've found receptors in most.

Chickens and chimps. Cats and carp. Pigeons and people.

So far, the only group that's missing is insects. For some reason, a broad swath of the animal life on earth doesn't seem to have the ability to make or use endocannabinoids. Nor do they respond to external cannabinoids. That is, everybody can get stoned, except insects.

We know this because of some painstaking work done by a group of researchers in New Zealand, who methodically cut up and pureed various part of insects, looking for endocannabinoid receptors.[3] If this sounds like a thankless job, you're right. Because they found approximately nothing.

First up: fruit flies (*Drosophila melanogaster*). Nope.

Next: honeybees (*Apis mellifera*). Nothing.

Then the water-strider (*Aquarius remigis,* formerly *Gerris remigis*). Sorry.

And, finally, a rather menacing black beetle (*Zophobas atratus*). Zero.

That absence of receptors is particularly interesting because in other respects, insects closely resemble us, at least with respect to their neurotransmitters. These little critters have a lot of neurotransmitters that we have, such as histamine, norepinephrine, and serotonin, just to name a few. So our neural chemistries actually have a lot in common. And yet our insect cousins seem to be missing these cannabinoid receptors and thus the ability to get buzzed.

Granted, there are a lot of insects out there. So the lack of endocannabinoid receptors in a handful isn't conclusive. But remember that researchers have had no trouble finding receptors in everything from sea urchins to chimpanzees. And striking out on four insects in a row suggests that our insect cousins who wandered off on that limb of the evolutionary tree left their endocannabinoids behind.

For the rest of us, though, there are a lot of animals with these receptors. That means that there are many animals that could potentially respond to endocannabinoids like anandamide. Or to THC or CBD. And that, in turn, means a lot of potential for research.

Noses and Nasturtiums

The discovery of endocannabinoids changed the way that many researchers thought about marijuana. Once they knew that there is a system of endocannabinoids across species, they began to think about other effects that molecules like THC and CBD might have.

The next logical step was to try to figure out what these endocanna-binoids do. And one of the simplest ways to figure out what a receptor does is to modify it. Just tweak is so it works a little differently. Or *really* tweak it so it doesn't work at all. Then step back and see what happens.

It's a little like tinkering with a car's engine. If you're not sure what that little round plastic thing next to the battery does, just take it out. Then try to start the car.

That may be pretty simple to do underneath a car's hood, but it's hard to do in a cell. In order to tweak a receptor, you need to know how it's constructed and where its gene sits on a chromosome. Then you need to be able to modify the gene, or make a different one from scratch. That's time-consuming and difficult.

Fortunately, there's an easier way to find out how changes to our can-nabinoid receptors affect how they work. Let those changes come to you.

Endocannabinoid receptors are encoded by genes, and genes vary among individuals and populations. Just as you and I both have noses, yours and mine are probably different sizes, different shapes, and have a different propensity to sneeze in response to a proffered bouquet of nasturtiums.

In the same way, endocannabinoid receptors vary. Sure, they have the same basic structure and function, just as noses do. But there can be a lot of differences among people. Scientists call these differences poly-morphisms.

You can think of each polymorphism as a small-scale experiment that can help us understand what cannabinoid receptors do. For in-stance, if we know that one person has a particular version of the CB1 receptor, we can see how that person is different from other people who carry other versions. In particular, if we know that people with one ver-sion of that receptor are more (or less) prone to a particular illness, then it's possible that endocannabinoids are somehow involved in that ill-ness. It's also possible, therefore, that THC or CBD or other cannabi-noids might be useful in treating that illness.

Several illnesses of this type are ones that you'd expect, because they're related to the way the brain works. For instance, certain variants of the CB1 receptor that appear on neurons in the brain are associated with a higher risk of developing attention deficit hyperactivity disorder (ADHD), and also post-traumatic stress disorder (PTSD).[4] Receptor gene variants might also affect our risk of drug dependency and depression.[5]

More surprising, perhaps, is the possibility that these receptors may be linked to other conditions that are at least partly outside the brain, such as obesity.[6] Even more surprising is the finding that conditions that have nothing to do with the brain (as far as we know) are associated with variants of the CB1 receptor. For instance, certain configurations of the CB1 receptors seem to be associated with a higher risk of osteoporosis.[7] So if CB1 receptors are implicated in these diseases, then maybe—just maybe—THC or CBD or other drugs that bind to those receptors might have a role in their treatment.

Lost in Translation

How could the CB1 and CB2 receptors be involved in such a wide variety of illnesses? Depression? PTSD? Obesity? Osteoporosis? It seems impossible that the natural endocannabinoids like anandamide and 2-AG that are designed to bind to these receptors could have so many effects.

Actually, it makes a lot of sense. Consider the word *den*. In English, it means "an animal's living room." But in German, *den* means "the." (Also, oddly, in Swahili.) In Dutch, a *den* is a pine tree. In Czech, it means "day." In Maori and Hindi and Georgian, *den* doesn't mean much of anything, as far as I know.

So what a word means depends on where you are and who you're talking to. That's hardly news to experienced travelers, who know the dangers of language that's lost in translation. Say the wrong thing to the wrong person and you might wind up in jail, or married.

Just as a single word or sound can have different meanings in different countries, cannabinoids like THC and CBD have different effects on their receptors, depending on where in the body those receptors are located.

For example, take CB1 receptors. They exist in neurons in the brain and they also exist in the liver. But they have vastly different effects in each of those places.[8]

In the brain, CB1 receptors appear in neurons. So a cannabinoid that binds to the CB1 receptor opens potassium channels and closes calcium channels. The result is the release of neurotransmitters that would make you feel high.

On the other hand, in the liver, there are no neurons with neurotransmitters to be released. Because . . . you're in the liver. And livers, generally speaking, don't get stoned. Instead, CB1 receptors in the liver increase fat storage. Same endocannabinoid, same receptor. But an entirely different result.

The Science of Keys and Locks

Why would our bodies rely on a handful of neurotransmitters and receptors to do so many things? And how could the THC and CBD in marijuana possibly be helpful if they have so many effects? This is a problem that makes an appearance in a famous joke by the comedian Steven Wright:

"One day, when I came home from work, I accidentally put my car key in the door of my apartment building. I turned it, and the whole building started up."

If you're not laughing, it's because you've never made this mistake. Also, perhaps, because text on a page doesn't do justice to Wright's deadpan—almost stoned—delivery. But the message is clear enough: put the wrong key in the wrong lock, and you might get a result that you didn't bargain for. That's as true for cannabinoids as it is for keys. And the results can be as confusing.

A substance like anandamide (or THC or CBD) exerts an effect wherever it ends up. In the liver, or in the brain, or anywhere else.

Wherever it is, as long as there are CB1 or CB2 receptors, it will do something.

And that raises a question: How is it that our bodies don't seem to be confounded by the fact that anandamide has divergent effects in different places?

Perhaps inevitably, the answer appears in another Steven Wright joke: A thermos is supposed to keep hot things hot and cold things cold. But how does it know?

A thermos doesn't have to "know," of course. And our cannabinoid receptors don't have to know, either. Just like that thermos, they work with what they have.

There are two basic kinds of hormones: those that act throughout the body and those that act in a specific, limited area. Endocrine hormones (like estrogen or insulin) are the ones that you're probably most familiar with. They're systemic, which means they act throughout the body. So parathyroid hormone, for instance, acts on the kidney and the gastrointestinal tract and on bone. Its effects are different in different organs, but those effects are all contributing toward the same goal of increasing blood levels of calcium.

Paracrine hormones, on the other hand, act locally. They have defined roles and narrow effects in certain parts of the body. For instance, paracrine hormones are sometimes produced in one cell and act on other cells that are right next door.

A prominent group of paracrine hormones are known as fibroblast growth factors. Basically, they're hormones that cause cells to grow, divide, and differentiate. So they must act locally. If you have a cut, you want the skin cells around that cut to grow. You definitely don't want that message to grow going out to all the cells in your body.

Endocannabinoids work as local paracrine hormones, and it seems that their production is often triggered when bad things happen. Specifically, cells use lipids that are in their membranes to produce endocannabinoids. That's neat, because this means they can do this on demand—quickly and easily. For instance, when a cell's calcium level rises, which often happens in response to stress, it can begin to produce endocannabinoids from its membrane.

So that's the rather elegant explanation of how one molecule can have so many different effects. How these receptors work, and what they do when they're activated, depends on where in the body they are located. This also explains why our endocannabinoid receptors are involved in so many different conditions, from obesity to depression.

That explanation answers one question, but it leads to another: If endocannabinoids like anandamide act locally, then what does marijuana do? The cannabinoids in a joint aren't local. Take a hit of a joint, and THC and CBD travel throughout your body.

This is a problem for anyone who wants to use medical marijuana, or its ingredients. Remember that in the brain, THC causes neurotransmitter release. In the liver, it increases fat stores. So if you disseminate THC throughout the body, for instance, you'll get neurotransmitters in the brain and fat in the liver.

That's why researchers have been interested for a long time in developing drugs that mimic anandamide and THC in certain ways. That is, they've looked for drugs that act on receptors in only one part of the body. And, hopefully, where they can have only one effect.

Breaking Bad Comes to a Corner Store Near You

How well have scientists been able to hack the endocannabinoid system? It turns out that the answer to that question isn't in the laboratories of prestigious universities or pharmaceutical companies. Instead, the most up-to-date science of this field of synthetic cannabinoid research can be seen in a strip mall in a seedy neighborhood in southern New Jersey. Or so I've been told.

I have to admit, this particular establishment doesn't look like it's an outpost at the frontiers of cannabinoid science. I'm in a semiurban neighborhood that's a little rough around the edges, and this establishment's wide plate-glass windows have been plastered with dark plastic that's cracked and peeling. The jury-rigged privacy glass may be cheap, but it's effective. I can't see anything inside. But this is the future of cannabinoid research we're talking about here, so I go in.

A bell rings overhead, barely audible over the background music that sounds a little like the soundtrack of a very bad dream, playing underwater. The floor is cheap linoleum, the ceiling is low particleboard, and the shelves all around me are stocked with enough drug paraphernalia to give all of the parents in New Jersey a collective panic attack.

There's a man behind the counter to my left who seems like he might be of help. He's in his twenties, with blond dreadlocks and a scruffy beard. He's wearing a raggedy rough-knit fisherman's sweater despite the room's warmth and the space heater crouched at his feet.

Unfortunately, he seems absorbed in a tattered copy of *A Wrinkle in Time*. I clear my throat. Finally, he looks up, and I tell him what I'm looking for: synthetic cannabinoids.

The dull look I receive in response suggests that this question has missed its mark. I try again.

Herbal marijuana?

His eyes light up and he nods.

"In back."

Indeed, at the very rear of the dim store, on a rack of shelves maybe 4 feet high and 6 feet wide, there are rows and rows of foil pouches. This is it. This is what I've been looking for. This could be the next big breakthrough in the science of medical marijuana.

I choose one package at random. It's called SOMA, and the label boasts that it's "a divine experience of body, mind & spirit." The letters in the name are spelled out by oddly shaped cartoon mushrooms that are wearing the white-spotted caps of *Amanita muscaria*.

What's in the package? The ingredient list is somewhat vague. There is *Amanita muscaria* extract. Also "herbal extracts, resins, and oils."

I try a few more packages, some of which are more forthcoming about their ingredients. There's *Salvia divinorum* ("diviner's sage"), for instance. It's a plant that grows in Mexico and contains psychoactive substances, including salvinorin A, which binds to kappa opioid and dopamine receptors in the brain.

And there's *Mitragyna speciosa*. Commonly known as Kratom (also kratum or ketum), it comes from a bush that is native to Southeast Asia. It's particularly interesting to me as a hospice physician because it contains chemicals that seem to bind to mu opioid receptors—the receptors on which medications like morphine act.

And there's *Leonotis leonurus*. It's known as lion's tail or wild dagga and grows in southern Africa, where it's been used as a sort of home-grown version of marijuana.

I'm reading these out loud—*Salvia divinorum, Mitragyna speciosa, Leonotis leonurus*—saying them softly to myself in hopes of remembering them. As I do, I realize that I sound like a first-year student at Hogwarts. (If you're alone as you're reading this, try it, you'll see what I mean.)

The legality of many of these herbs is hotly debated. They're widely available in some countries and more restricted in others. However, the Internet has democratized availability, and virtually anyone with on-line access can procure them.

There are other herbs listed on the packages, too. But just herbs. Alas, that's all that's in these packages. The labels are stridently clear about this.

"No additives!" one promises.

"Nothing artificial!"

Just herbs. But herbs are not what I'm looking for.

As I told the guy at the front of the store, I'm looking for synthetic cannabinoids. And the easiest place to find them is in packages like these. Even in places where marijuana is illegal, these synthetics are often unregulated, and so they're added to herbs, giving a wide range of psychoactive effects.

Researchers have been creating synthetic cannabinoids in test tubes for the past fifty years, and those experiments have turned out hundreds of them, which fall into several families. There are the JWH cannabinoids, developed by a chemist named John W. Huffman who used to work at Clemson University. There's another family, labeled CP, which were created by chemists at Pfizer in the 1970s. And Alexandros Makriyannis at Northeastern University has several molecules to his credit, which are known by the prefix AM. Those that were developed at Hebrew University by Raphael Mechoulam's group are labeled with an "HU." (Synthetics from a fifth, unnamed, family are known simply, and rather boringly, for their chemical structure: benzoylindoles.)

Many of these synthetics have appeared in herbal marijuana products, like those on the back shelves of this head shop. However, few have had their therapeutic benefits rigorously tested in people. So herbal marijuana packages like these generally go out of their way to claim that they don't contain such "additives."

In fact, only one synthetic has made it past all of the considerable hurdles of drug testing. That was the brainchild of Louis Lemberger. He used to be a scientist at the National Institutes of Health, but then he went to work for Eli Lilly in 1971. When he got there, he developed the drug nabilone, which is used for the treatment of nausea with chemotherapy.[9]

But Lemberger didn't just want to create a synthetic that was useful for nausea. He also wanted to create a synthetic that didn't make people high.

You could argue that that's a rather silly goal. For many of my patients struggling through chemotherapy and nausea while fighting a potentially lethal cancer, a little euphoria would be welcome. But Lemberger and his colleagues knew that the key to marketing a synthetic was to delete that stoned feeling. At least at the right doses. So they were no doubt elated—even euphoric—when they found that they had been successful in eliminating most of the psychoactive effects of their new drug.[10]

Nabilone does cause some euphoria, though. We know this because of another study in which researchers gave nabilone, THC, and a placebo to experienced marijuana users. Those subjects—who knew a lot about feeling stoned—thought that nabilone was very different from a placebo, and not so different from THC.[11] That is, they were impressed by nabilone in ways that Lemberger and colleagues probably would have preferred that they weren't.

Still, nabilone is an intriguing example of what might be possible someday. Although it does have some psychoactive effects, those effects have been attenuated. And it does relieve nausea. So that's preliminary evidence that it might be possible to design versions of THC or CBD that offer more of the effects people want, with fewer effects that drug companies don't want.

Many of the synthetics that have been created are probably represented in this particular business establishment. However, it seems that something has been lost in translation. The packages I see around me have names like *Black Mamba* or *Sky Mamba* or *OMG, Hysteria, Bizarro,* and *No Joke.* They sport lurid packages that remind me more than a little of pulp fiction cover art of the bodice-ripping variety. For instance, there's a sinister orange eye on one (*Spice Gold*). Another features a picture of what appears to be an ostrich in a top hat (*Neon Circus*). That's about par for the course.

But it's pretty obvious that whoever is marketing this stuff is spending all of their capital on artwork. The packaging is amateurish, to say the least. But it's also been vetted by lawyers. One offers this disclaimer: "Does not mimick [*sic*] THC."

Well, if these substances don't mimic THC, what exactly do they do?

I pick up the package with the well-dressed ostrich and I take it up to the counter, where the guy is, if anything, even less helpful than he was five minutes ago. I ask him if this, um, herbal product has any medical uses.

His blank look tells me pretty much everything I need to know about his thoughts on the subject. He pauses to think for a moment.

"It's . . . you know . . . chilling."

Could they have medical uses? Could they help people?

"Why not? Anything's possible, man."

I thank him, put the formally dressed ostrich back in his place, and head for the door.

Even if the guy behind the counter of that head shop doesn't know it, we've come a long way from the discovery of THC and CBD. In theory, at least, it should be possible to design cannabinoids that have very specific effects. Relief of back pain without hallucinations? Sure. Nausea relief with just a little bit of euphoria? OK.

If the last fifty years are any indication, these efforts might very well succeed. In a relatively short period of time, science has made enormous progress. Not only have researchers isolated the bliss molecule, its receptors, and natural molecules like THC and CBD, they've also created dozens of synthetics with a wide range of properties.

Who knows what could be possible? It seems likely that someday we'll have drugs that target endocannabinoid receptors in various parts of the body. And perhaps we'll even have drugs that can be tailored to some of the more common receptor polymorphisms that exist, so that treatment can be tailored not only to a particular symptom, but also to a patient's genetic makeup.

That's actually some of the most interesting science of marijuana. True, it's a long way from bongs and joints. And still hypothetical. But, in the wise words of that head shop clerk, anything's possible.

Don't Mess with Mr. Smiley

Before we get too excited about the future of synthetic cannabinoids, though, there's one problem we'll need to deal with. And it might be a big one.

The good news is that you can't fatally overdose on marijuana. There don't seem to be any CB1 or CB2 receptors in the brain stem, which controls important functions like breathing. So in theory, even massive amounts of marijuana shouldn't cause a fatal overdose in the same way that too much morphine would, for instance. That makes marijuana safer than other drugs like morphine in an overdose.

But we don't know whether these synthetic cannabinoids play by the same rules. They are drugs that have been created in laboratories. We have no idea what receptors they might bind to, or what they might do.

Are they as safe as marijuana is? It depends on whom you ask. According to the mother of Nicholas Colbert, the answer is a resounding "no."

Colbert's story has brought me to South Chelton Road, a wide street that cuts roughly north-south through Colorado Springs. At least in this neighborhood, South Chelton is lined with low-rise apartments that look clean and neatly kept. In a small strip mall on the east side of the street, there's a row of vacant storefronts, a pizza place, a discount Cricket cell phone store, a 7-Eleven, and a Kwik Mart convenience store. It's not the sort of place you'd expect to produce a wrongful death lawsuit. But a wrongful death is exactly what the mother of Nicholas Colbert alleges happened here.[12]

I park my rental car and make my way through the nearly empty parking lot to the Kwik Mart. The store is small, clean, and well lighted.

Over there is the counter where, late on the night of September 20, 2011, Colbert purchased a small jar of so-called synthetic marijuana. A few minutes earlier, he said good night to his mother, telling her he was going out to get some smokes. Then he drove here. The product he bought that night, according to the lawsuit, was sold under the brand name "Mr. Smiley."

Shortly thereafter, the lawsuit alleges, Mr. Colbert smoked a quantity of the product, and died suddenly. His mother, Stephane Colbert, found him dead in their home on September 21. He had been in excellent health, the lawsuit notes, and there is no reason to believe that his death was caused by anything other than what he smoked that night.[13]

The lawsuit also alleges that two Kwik Mart employees, Alex Lee and Sung Soo Lee, sold Mr. Smiley several times, despite the statewide ban on the product that was imposed in March of 2011. The lawsuit also alleges that the employees would counsel customers on its use, recommending techniques for smoking it.

As evidence, the lawsuit cites the finding in Mr. Colbert's autopsy of two synthetics: JWH-018 and AM-2201.

The initials JWH tell us that JWH-018 is one of the family of synthetic cannabinoids created in John W. Huffman's lab at Clemson University, as mentioned above. It acts at both CB1 and CB2 receptors and, like many synthetics, has been found to cause anxiety, agitation, confusion, and seizures. Also, like many synthetics, it is considerably more potent than THC.

AM-2201 is one of the compounds discovered by Alexandros

Makriyannis at Northeastern University. Its properties are less well described, but it seems to have many of the same effects as its better-
known cousin JWH-018.

I cruise the aisles quickly, looking for anything resembling Mr. Smiley. There's milk. And potato chips. M&M's. Beef jerky. There are cigarettes and cigars behind the counter, but that's about it. I see no signs of
any synthetic marijuana.

Besides the risk of overdose, another problem with synthetics has to
do with the way that the body's receptors bind to many of them. We're
learning that the receptor binding process is different for many synthetics than it is for, say, THC.

Imagine these molecules are like customers at a taco truck. Some
molecules, like THC, are agonists. They just walk up and place an order. Others, like CBD, are partial agonists. They take their sweet time,
and slow the line down for everyone else.

But many of the synthetics are very aggressive agonists. They crash
their way to the front of the line, elbowing other molecules out of the
way. Then they reach in and grab what they want. If you're using a synthetic for the first time, and you're expecting the dose of an average
joint, you could be very surprised.

In fact, both of the synthetics implicated in Nicholas Colbert's death,
JWH-018 and AM-2201, are full agonists. This makes them much more
potent than THC. Indeed, AM-2201 in particular can be active at doses
of only half a milligram, compared with usual doses of 10 to 20 milligrams for THC. So even small amounts could have unexpected and
dangerous effects.

For instance, another death apparently occurred when a victim
passed out in a hot tub and drowned.[14] Even though it's not precisely
true to say that a synthetic caused that man's death directly (for instance, by a heart attack or cardiac arrhythmia), it's also pretty fair to
say that if he hadn't passed out, he would probably still be alive.

That brings us to a third concern with synthetics: side effects. Mostly,
we just don't know what other side effects they might cause. Even if they
don't bind to receptors in the brain stem and can't cause you to stop

breathing, they could nevertheless cause other harms, most of which haven't been discovered yet.

Indeed, there are gruesome stories of rare but serious side effects. One person suffered a stroke that resulted from synthetic cannabinoids.[15] Another report describes a patient who developed diffuse inflammation and fluid in his lungs after smoking synthetics, requiring more than a week in an intensive care unit.[16] And there are numerous reports of various other forms of adverse reactions such as hallucinations, nausea, vomiting, chest pain, and seizures.[17] Remember, too, that we all come equipped with different cannabinoid receptor polymorphisms. A molecule that does nothing to me might make you sleepy, or confused, or agitated.

The results of the Colbert lawsuit haven't been reported as of early 2015, so we don't know whether a court agreed that Mr. Smiley was to blame for Nicholas Colbert's death. Scientifically, we'll never know. But given how complex the endocannabinoid system is, and how little we know about the effects of synthetics like JWH-018, it seems plausible to me that whatever was in that package Colbert bought at the Kwik Mart could have contributed to his death.

At the very least, synthetic cannabinoids should come with a warning, at least for recreational use. Many should be banned altogether.

Indeed, no less an expert than John W. Huffman is quoted as saying in a radio interview that the recreational use of synthetic cannabinoids has turned out to be "dangerous."[18] In fact, many are illegal in the United States and in other countries. But there are a lot of synthetics, and creative entrepreneurs have proved clever at keeping one step ahead of the law, often substituting a new synthetic to replace one that has been banned.

But Huffman is also philosophical about his role in all of this. He developed these synthetics for scientific purposes. Much of his research was funded by highly competitive grants from the National Institutes of Health. As for the people who have made money by manufacturing and marketing compounds like JWH-018, he says, "You can't be responsible for what idiots are going to do."

Nevertheless, we're not talking about recreational use. We're talking about developing synthetics with specific properties, for very particular uses. Nabilone is the first example to be used clinically, but it certainly won't be the last.

The Grandfather of Medical Marijuana

Risks aside, will we ever be able to use synthetics and the endocannabinoid system to help people? To answer that question, I decide to talk to one person who knows more about marijuana research and its future than anyone else: Raphael Mechoulam, the grandfather of medical marijuana.

In a stairwell outside his laboratory at Hebrew University in Jerusalem, I'm staring at what seems to be a pretty comprehensive collection of various herbs and plants that have been used for medicinal purposes over the years. Glass-fronted racks are crammed with bottles and jars with glass stoppers and carefully printed, yellowing labels. There is *Cinchona succirubra*, for instance. That's the source of quinine, an antimalarial. And *Digitalis lanata* (the original source of digitalis, used for heart disease). And, oddly, *Satureja thymbra*, which as far as I know is useful mostly as a flavoring for soups and stews.

There's a rather important plant that's missing. And it's a particularly odd omission, if you consider that I'm standing outside Mechoulam's laboratory. On second thought, I can see why someone known for studying illicit substances would not want to put a stash of his research material in an unlocked display case.

But where is the man? I wander around a ring of laboratories and offices, populated by remarkably young, attractive, and hip technicians and graduate students. What is most noticeable, though, is how unfailingly polite they are. One thin, bearded young man, perhaps aware of the implications of a stranger wandering aimlessly through a lab that studies cannabinoids, strips off his gloves and escorts me to Mechoulam's office, where he deposits me with a soft-spoken "all the best."

Raphael Mechoulam greets me cordially, ushering me into his office. Its dimensions are modest, especially considering that this entire floor of laboratory space (and the glass case outside) is the product of more than fifty years of his work. Lined with bookshelves, his office is surprisingly neat.

Mechoulam is in his eighties, but he speaks and moves quickly, almost impatiently. He's balding, with a snow-white ring of remaining hair that frames an active, intelligent face. A blue button-down shirt and brown trousers hang loosely on a spare frame.

"So. What questions do you have for me?"

What I really want him to tell me about is the future of medical marijuana. I want to know what Mechoulam thinks about what's going on now, and what might someday be possible. And so I start by telling him about Caleb, the man with metastatic cancer I met in the first chapter. What does he think about the widespread welcome that medical marijuana has received lately?

"I'm not sure that I'm very happy with it," he says slowly. "Now it's big business. It's not being analyzed. People get one thing today and another thing tomorrow." He pauses, looking hard at a spot about 6 inches above my head.

"That's not the way to do medicine. The doctor tells you to take this, in this amount, in such and such a way. Everything people get should be well defined and well analyzed. At the moment, it's a mess. And I'm not happy with it."

There's not nearly enough clinical research, he tells me. Good research, using cannabinoids in defined amounts.

"And the studies—good studies. So very, very few. Quite frankly, that's outrageous. If you have so many people using it, there should be clinical evidence."

He's particularly dismissive of many studies that test the effects of smoking natural marijuana buds, or other natural marijuana-derived products. He points out that usually there's no chemical analysis or quality control.

"Pharmacologists—serious pharmacologists—won't work with a

mixture," Mechoulam says. "They want to know exactly what one is putting into an experiment."

And that's pretty much impossible if what you're putting into an experiment is simply the contents of something you harvested from your garden, dried, and pulverized. Instead, Mechoulam would like to see more research on THC, CBD, and other cannabinoids.

Think about that *Cinchona succirubra* in the display case outside Mechoulam's office. The bark of the chinchona tree was used back in the sixteenth century as a treatment for malaria. Back then it was little more than herbal medicine. But then someone figured out how to extract the active ingredient in reliable concentrations, with dependable properties. That's quinine, which is still used as an antimalarial.

Mechoulam thinks that the science of marijuana isn't yet at that stage. "People use marijuana once, it works. Second time, no. They don't have the same dose. They're not getting the same drug." He shakes his head in frustration.

Mechoulam is referring to a common criticism of medical marijuana that I've witnessed in my research for this book. When the THC and CBD content of marijuana varies between buds, some people may not be getting an adequate dose. And there are safety concerns, too, since some people may be getting more psychoactive THC than they need.

Above all, Mechoulam says, it's about the patient. "And you don't want to disappoint a patient, do you? First, you help them. Then not. Then where the hell are you?"

If Mechoulam isn't impressed by the current state of the science of medical marijuana, is he hopeful about its future? He's been in this field longer than anyone else. He's seen it mature into a science of synthetic chemistry, genetics, and neuroscience. So I ask him where he thinks the science of cannabinoids is going to go next.

Raphael Mechoulam is very interested, first, in the role that CBD could play in modulating inflammation. In fact, he's begun to think of CBD as part of a global "protective system" that controls potentially harmful inflammation in the body. That could have implications for all sorts of conditions, including autoimmune disorders. So I can see why he's so enthusiastic.

And, as we've seen before, CBD might have a starring role here, too. So far, most of what we know about CBD and arthritis comes from laboratory studies, but what we know is very interesting. For instance, in one study,[19] Mechoulam and his collaborators induced an inflammatory arthritis in mice by injecting them with collagen. That provoked their immune systems to react to their native collagen, causing an inflammatory arthritis of the sort that occurs in diseases like rheumatoid arthritis or lupus. They found that CBD effectively reduced inflammation, immune cell activation, and blood levels of inflammatory cytokines such as tumor necrosis factor. For what it's worth, that study also describes the mice's "clinical" improvement, although the report is a little vague about what that looks like.

Even more interesting is a study of 169 people, some of whom had been using marijuana regularly, which found that users had significantly lower levels of the inflammatory molecule interleukin 6 (IL-6).[20] IL-6 is another cytokine, and is typically elevated in diseases like rheumatoid arthritis. So if it's lower in chronic marijuana users, cannabinoids might have a long-term ability to curb the body's inflammatory response.

Mechoulam is also interested in the role that cannabinoids might play in epigenetics, or how the body regulates the expression of genes. He describes the way that enzymes increase or decrease a gene's activity, or turn it on or off. Cannabinoids might affect that process.

"In one case," he says, "anandamide has been shown to regulate DNA. And CBD does this for a skin disease—psoriasis. If that's true, it may be involved in regulation of DNA. Maybe that's why cannabinoids are involved in so many systems."

This is one of the most interesting things I've heard in our conversation so far. It means that the effects of cannabinoids might not be limited to their effects on receptors. They might also play a much more fundamental role, by influencing which genes our bodies choose to pay attention to.

"This is not working on symptoms of disease," he says enthusiastically, his hands gesturing expressively as he speaks. "Now this is working on the *basis* of disease."

Will that be successful? Mechoulam isn't certain. But he's hopeful that science will make progress in his lifetime. The methods are known, he points out. And the science is there. "It is certainly possible."

There's a third area of research that Mechoulam would like very much to see. But he talks about it wistfully. He's not sure how to begin to conceptualize it.

"Cannabinoids," he says, "may have something to do with our psychology and personality." He looks at me appraisingly. "Why are you and I so different?"

Fortunately that seems to be a rhetorical question.

"It's possible that these compounds have something to do with it. Maybe yes, maybe no." He shrugs. "But we should find out."

And will we?

He tells me that he's optimistic about discoveries related to inflammation and epigenetics, but then he's silent for a moment. "The psychology thing, I'm not sure. Most certainly I'm not going to do it. I'm an old man. One has to realize what one can do, and what one has to leave to others."

Then he asks me, more or less out of the blue, how old I am.

I tell him. (He's just that sort of guy.)

He thinks for a second, then he points out that he's forty years older than I am.

"The basic problem is that kind of research takes many years. And I don't have too many years."

But he still has plenty of time. As he walks me to the door, he continues to talk about research he is doing and more that he wants to do. He keeps adding to his list of people I should talk with and questions I should be asking.

We really need more clinical trials, he says. "Until we have more clinical trials, the field will be kind of . . . marginal for most doctors. You are serious people. You ask where's the meat? In many cases we don't have the meat."

But—and I can't believe I'm asking this—will we ever have the meat?

"Oh yes. It will take time. But yes."

Outside Mechoulam's laboratory, standing in front of the display cases, I have one more question, although it doesn't have much to do with the science of cannabinoids. But it's a question that's been nagging at me.

Raphael Mechoulam and Bill Devane used a little poetic license in naming the molecule anandamide. They used the Sanskrit word *ananda*, or "bliss." I'm curious why they chose Sanskrit, rather than, say, Hebrew.

He tells me that Bill Devane, the leader of that study, was studying Sanskrit at the time. Since they were in Israel, of course they did look for a Hebrew alternative, but couldn't find one. There are a lot of words for sorrow in Hebrew, he points out, but there aren't many for joy.

The Future of Medical Marijuana

If there's one thing I've learned about the future of medical marijuana, it's that the future—whatever it is—will be much broader and more complex than smoking a joint. As we've seen, researchers are just beginning to understand the function of cannabinoid receptors. And we're still in the very early stages of figuring out what those receptors do, and how to take advantage of them to treat symptoms and cure disease.

So it's difficult to predict where the science of marijuana might take us. Even the next few years are uncertain. But with Mechoulam's speculations in mind, I can offer a couple of suggestions.

First, I'm guessing that there will be a lot of interest in testing synthetic cannabinoids. There are dozens of new molecules that have been developed already, and there are more on the way. Some have made an appearance in "herbal marijuana," but we don't know much about what these synthetics do, or how they might be helpful. It seems possible—even likely—that some of them offer benefits that we haven't discovered yet.

Second, there are a lot of natural cannabinoids that appear in marijuana in small amounts. I've told you what we know about THC and CBD, but they're just the most prominent cannabinoids. And just as we'll learn more about synthetics, we'll probably also learn a lot about what these other cannabinoids can do.

It's the third prediction that's most speculative and most exciting. Mechoulam talked about the role of cannabinoids in inflammation, in epigenetics, and even in human personality. He was suggesting that we should be thinking about marijuana not as a medicine, but as a doorway to a very complex system. He's suggesting that what's interesting is not so much what marijuana does, but what it tells us about the way that our bodies work.

To understand what that might mean, think about the vitamin D that's used to fortify milk. Vitamin D was first discovered in cod liver oil, which was observed to cure stunted bone growth (rickets) in children. But there's more.

Vitamin D turned out to be important not only because it cures rickets, but also because it led to discoveries of how calcium metabolism works, and how bones are formed and remodeled. (One such discovery was that vitamin D isn't really a vitamin, but rather a hormone.) That is, the vitamin D in cod liver oil was a very crude way to hack into the body's system of calcium and bones, paving the way for research that's brought us treatments for bone fractures, cancer metastases in bone, and osteoporosis in older adults.

When scientists figured out that vitamin D was responsible for bone formation, we were able to learn about the rest of that system. We discovered other hormones, for instance, such as parathyroid hormone, which regulate calcium. And we began to map out the extent of that system, which spans multiple organ systems, including the liver and the kidneys. We've learned all of that from the simple observation that cod liver oil is good for bone formation.

In much the same way, the observation that marijuana might be useful in treating pain or seizures may be only a very small first step in unraveling the science of the endocannabinoid system. Just as vitamin D proved to be only a part of our bodies' system of calcium metabolism, it seems possible that THC and CBD are only a small part of what our endocannabinoid system can do. They may be effective in treating insomnia or seizures, and that would be worth celebrating, of course. But they might also be the leading edge of a new world of science.

That's what Mechoulam is hoping. He's not just studying marijuana, or its ingredients. At least, that's not his ultimate aim. He's really interested in how those molecules and their effects point to new discoveries that could be much bigger, and more far-reaching, than anything we've seen so far. Not content to think just about symptoms, he wants to be able to shape personality, control inflammation, tweak the immune system, and—maybe—cure cancer.

10

A Long Strange Trip

Archie Bunker and "Medical" Marijuana

"Ohhh, so now pot's a 'medicine,' right? Now they're handing out *pre-scriptions*? You gotta be kidding me!"

I'm in a taxi driven by an irascible guy who looks like he's about fifty and has been driving a cab for pretty much that whole time. I'm guessing he's constructed his moral worldview by watching Archie Bunker on *All in the Family* reruns. He's wrestling the cab through New York traffic with the finesse of a matador and the impassivity of the dictator of a small Latin American country.

When I climbed in at Penn Station, I made the mistake of telling Archie that I was going to meet a researcher who studies medical marijuana. The result has been a twenty-minute tirade that has been by turns vituperative, dismissive, and caustic. Also wildly entertaining.

But it's been difficult to figure out what his stance on marijuana is. He's not against it per se. Certainly he's not morally opposed. It's more that he thinks the whole idea is a grand joke.

"Sick people getting stoned? Hey, why not? And why stop with marijuana? Why not try LSD?" If your reality really sucks, he says several times, why not get as far away from it as you can?

As I'm listening to this free-association rant, keeping an eye out for the bumpers of other cars, I'm having two reactions more or less simultaneously.

First, what I'm hearing sounds eerily familiar. The opinions that Archie is spouting are pretty much what I was saying a year ago when I first started this project. In fact, I'm pretty sure that if Archie and I had met a year ago, we would have shared a good laugh about the grand joke of "medical" marijuana.

But it's my second reaction that surprises me: I find myself disagreeing. I find myself wanting to argue. With a New York City cabdriver. I should state for the record that this is not something that I have ever been inspired to do before.

Marijuana does offer benefits, I tell him during one of his brief pauses for breath. I was surprised, too, I say mildly. It's useful in treating certain types of pain, like—

But Archie isn't listening. He's off and running again, talking about how people these days are coddled, about how they want everything handed to them. How getting high is just getting high, it's not *treating* anything.

We slice across three lanes of traffic, cutting off a bicycle messenger, a bus, and a delivery van, and screech to a halt in the general vicinity of the curb. I pay him, backing out of earshot as fast as I can. As I turn to make my escape, Archie is still ranting about Obamacare and the DEA and—for reasons that are best left to the imagination—Girl Scouts.

The Blacksmith and the Boxer

It's been a year since I met Caleb, the blacksmith whose trip across the country in search of medical marijuana prompted my own journey to figure out what this stuff is and what it does. In that time, I've talked with dozens of experts, patients, and activists. I've slogged through hundreds of studies of marijuana. I can even say that I've had some limited experience with its effects on me (and on my patio furniture).

Along the way, I've graduated from a hard-nosed skepticism to an open-mindedness that I never would have believed possible a year ago. That shift has been the result of the people I've met and the stories I've heard. Especially Caleb's.

In fact, I've often thought about Caleb because I've realized that although his story is unusual, the challenges he faced aren't unique. He's a guy who figured out through trial and error that marijuana was the only thing that helped him. And yet he couldn't get it.

He could get morphine. And benzodiazepines. In fact, he had a stash collecting dust in the back of a cupboard. He could have gotten other drugs, too, if he'd been willing to take them.

But he was convinced that only marijuana helped him, and he survived from day to day with what little marijuana he could borrow or buy. That seems like a powerful argument that we should take medical marijuana seriously.

Is Marijuana a Medicine?

So: Does marijuana work?

Well, one thing I've learned is that this isn't the right question to ask.

Does a hammer work? Sure, if you want to pound a nail. But if you want to fix a frozen iPhone, not so much. So whether marijuana "works" depends on what you want it to do.

Marijuana seems to be quite effective in treating neuropathic pain, and maybe ordinary, nociceptive pain, too. Or maybe not. But I wouldn't be surprised if it does turn out to be useful for nociceptive pain. A lot of pain is caused by, or exacerbated by, inflammation. And we know that cannabinoids have anti-inflammatory properties, much as drugs like ibuprofen do.

It definitely works for nausea. It probably improves appetite, too, even if it may not help people to gain weight. It's probably useful for insomnia, although we don't know for sure. And it might be helpful in managing the symptoms of anxiety and PTSD.

Then there are uses that are still hypothetical. Like treating the symptoms of dementia or Parkinson's disease, or as a complement to exposure therapy for PTSD. I can't imagine telling Archie the cabdriver about those uses, because they're still just ideas. But the evidence we have is promising.

Another potential use I decided not to mention during that cab ride was curing cancer. Probably all we can say right now is that maybe, someday, we'll have evidence either way, although, like Donald Abrams, the San Francisco oncologist, I'm both worried and sad when I hear people bragging that they've forsworn chemotherapy and are instead relying solely on marijuana.

If marijuana is effective in relieving some symptoms—or at least is as effective as other medications—then is it safe?

Well, maybe. Although I've been impressed by marijuana's benefits, I've been surprised by its risks. And there are lots of them.

When I began this journey, I figured that marijuana was unlikely to do any real harm. Aside from the obvious risks of serious injury and property damage associated with operating a vehicle while under the influence, I assumed that marijuana was pretty benign.

Here, too, I was wrong. The risks of addiction, for instance, seem to be substantial. Then there are the risks of psychosis and (perhaps) of schizophrenia. Add in the potential for heart attacks or stroke, too. There are still many other risks, and even if those risks are small and uncertain, their results could be devastating and perhaps even fatal.

Granted, those risks are trivial for someone like Caleb, whose cancer is likely to end his life very soon. But for many of the other patients I've met—many in their thirties or even their twenties—any risks have a long time to play themselves out. So even small incremental risks that accumulate over years or decades are worth worrying about.

Where does that leave us? Is marijuana a medicine? A year ago, I found that idea as laughable as Archie does. Pot? A medicine? That proposal seemed as wishful and deluded as declaring single malt Scotch a medicine.

And I have to say I am still skeptical. Marijuana's ingredients aren't as refined and defined as the ingredients in a pill are. A joint is hardly a medicine.

Sure, there are efforts under way to standardize marijuana and its products. My visit to Cannlabs' basement testing facility is a testament to how far the industry has come. But even that lab only tests for some cannabinoids. The rest remain a mystery, and probably vary from plant to plant, and from gummy bear to gummy bear. That variability, it seems to me, makes it very difficult to call marijuana a "medicine" in the same way that, say, penicillin is a medicine.

One interesting exception is a drug like Sativex, the treatment for nausea. Sativex is the carefully calibrated mixture of THC and CBD that have been extracted from plants. It's a medicine that preserves at least some of the natural mixture of cannabinoids, making it closer to natural marijuana than, say, pure THC (e.g., dronabinol). But Sativex is an exception. Indeed, as of 2014 it wasn't even approved for use in the United States.

So most people are still using marijuana rather than drugs like Sativex or dronabinol. Or, increasingly, they're using marijuana-based products like oil or edibles. That will probably continue to be the most common form in which people get THC and CBD, because they don't require a doctor's prescription.

For those reasons, I still think of marijuana as more or less equivalent to an herbal remedy. It's essentially plant-based stuff with numerous active and inactive ingredients, only some of which we understand. And those ingredients make an appearance in varying doses and ratios among plants and between crops.

That's not a fatal flaw. In fact, there are plenty of herbal remedies that are widely used, and even recommended by doctors. For instance, people take echinacea for cold symptoms, black cohosh (*Actaea racemosa*) for perimenopausal symptoms, Gingko biloba extract to preserve memory, and Saint-John's-wort (*Hypericum perforatum*) for depression. Some are effective, and others are still a mystery. Nevertheless, the fact that they are plant extracts rather than compounds synthesized in a laboratory hasn't dampened enthusiasm for their use. So calling marijuana an herbal remedy is by no means an indictment.

Overall, as long as we think of marijuana as an herbal remedy, I've become a pretty strong believer. There's a caveat, though. And it's a big one.

Right now, we can say that marijuana and its ingredients are effective in treating some medical problems, because marijuana is as good as other prescription drugs. Or, at least, it's less toxic than those drugs are. That is, marijuana gets my vote of confidence for symptoms like neuropathic pain and nausea because for some patients it's better than the competition.

But the competition is getting better. Remember that marijuana was once used to treat glaucoma. It wasn't very effective, but it was better than other drugs that were available. Now, though, prescription drugs are much more effective than marijuana is, so marijuana is no longer recommended, although some people no doubt still use it.

I wouldn't be surprised if marijuana gets left behind in the same way for other symptoms. As we develop better drugs for pain and nausea and anxiety, for instance, it's possible that marijuana will look less impressive five years from now. Maybe better, safer drugs will put marijuana out of business.

Of course, it's also possible that marijuana will become more effective, too. As we learn more about its key ingredients, we might find ways to increase its usefulness. For instance, new delivery mechanisms like patches and better vape pens might help. Increasing marijuana's CBD content might be useful, too.

Nevertheless, it seems unlikely that these sorts of modest advances will keep marijuana relevant in the long run. The pharmaceutical industry has an enormous financial stake in developing drugs to treat common symptoms like pain or nausea or anxiety. And we're sure to see new and better drugs on the horizon. Even if marijuana's effectiveness increases a little, that won't be enough to keep pace with the efforts of a multibillion-dollar pharmaceutical industry.

That would be especially true if the pharmaceutical industry began to turn its attention to the endocannabinoid system. Raphael Mechoulam was optimistic about all of the ways in which that system might be harnessed—or "hacked"—to relieve symptoms and cure disease. It will take time, but the pharmaceutical industry will eventually figure out how to bypass the marijuana plant and develop drugs that work directly on our endocannabinoid receptors.

That's not to say that the medical marijuana industry will go up in smoke. Even as newer, better drugs are developed, marijuana will always have two key advantages. The first, obviously, is the fact that marijuana makes you feel good. Very few prescription drugs can make that claim now.

The second advantage for marijuana is subtler, but just as important. Lisa, the woman with lupus who introduced me to Sasha the Wonder Dog at the United Health and Wellness clinic, said that medical marijuana was the best thing that had ever happened to her because it gave her a sense of control. She could choose what she used, and when, and how. And she didn't need a prescription from a doctor, just a letter of recommendation. That sense of control, and the confidence that comes with it, is probably going to keep medical marijuana relevant, no matter how many other new drugs are developed.

Crowdsourced Science

I'm optimistic about the future of medical marijuana not only because of what we're learning, but also because of *how* we're learning it. Specifically, medical marijuana seems uniquely suited for a new brand of crowdsourced science. That's science by the people and for the people.

As an example, consider a paper that was published in 2014, around the time I was sitting in Raphael Mechoulam's laboratory in Jerusalem. It describes a modest little study that enrolled twenty-two patients with Parkinson's disease.[1] (As it did in Caleb's case, Parkinson's causes a wide range of symptoms, including muscle rigidity, resting tremor, and slowed movement.) This was an open-label study, so-called because the patients knew what they were getting, and their doctors did, too. The study found that after a single exposure to inhaled marijuana, patients' symptoms of muscle rigidity and tremor improved, and they were able to move more freely.

What's most fascinating about this study is not in its description of increased freedom of movement, which is very preliminary. In fact, another small study found that CBD improves quality of life in patients with Parkinson's, but doesn't appear to improve patients' ability to walk or move.[2] So we don't know whether marijuana is useful in treating Parkinson's.

The most important line in the paper describing this study is a brief one buried in its technical details. As they make the case for why their study is important, the investigators mention anecdotal evidence that marijuana might help with symptoms of Parkinson's. Specifically, they cite "media reports."

That caught my attention because the person responsible for those media reports is Zach Klein, the filmmaker in Tel Aviv who had administered medical marijuana to nursing home residents. In a scene from his marijuana documentary, a man who has suffered from Parkinson's for years can finally write his name. That emblematic image became the cornerstone of the film, and it also prompted these researchers to organize a study that produced results that were published in a legitimate medical journal.

The fact that those researchers found the inspiration for a study in a film isn't just life imitating art. It's part of a broader theme of scientists imitating people. It's crowdsourced science.

Barth Wilsey, the anesthesiologist who studied the effects of marijuana on neuropathic pain, said that he heard about marijuana's effect on neuropathic pain from the patients from Oakland whom he met during his fellowship in a pain clinic. And Orrin Devinsky, the neurologist at NYU Langone's epilepsy center who decided to do his trial of CBD for childhood seizures, embarked on that research at least in part because of the success stories that he was hearing from parents.

The Internet is becoming a powerful tool for people struggling with serious illnesses. Cal and Cindy learned about CBD oil from an online support group, for instance, and many of the patients I've met in researching this book turned to medical marijuana because of what they found online. Add in patient-centered websites such as PatientsLikeMe, an online information-sharing network, and you have a powerful set of tools to learn about medical marijuana's benefits and risks.

If I'm optimistic about the future of medical marijuana—and I am—it's because of the potential of crowdsourcing. Although they're no substitute for randomized controlled trials, those stories are nevertheless a quick way of figuring out what sorts of trials we should be doing. They can tell us which symptoms might respond, and what doses might be effective. Those stories can also give us hints of risks that might exist. Even now, before we have enough evidence from long-term studies, patient stories are telling us to beware of risks of addiction, heart attacks, and psychosis.

When we spoke in his pleasantly cluttered office at San Francisco General Hospital, Donald Abrams gently chided me for referring to the "field" of medical marijuana research, as if such a thing existed. He said that there weren't very many clinical researchers doing good work, and there wasn't much available funding, either. It was premature, he said, to refer to a field of medical marijuana research in the same way that we refer to a field of, say, pain research. And I admit he's right.

But even if there isn't yet a field of research focused on the clinical use of medical marijuana, there is a crowd. A big one. And it's a crowd that, by and large, is more connected than most.

So we have lots of people who are trying marijuana in various ways, for a wide variety of indications. Sometimes it will work, and sometimes it won't. And, if we're being honest, sometimes people will *think* that it works but will be fooled by the placebo effect.

Nevertheless, we can harness these thousands of little experiments going on every day. We can get a sense of what might work and what probably won't work. And—what is probably just as important—we can learn about whether marijuana is safe.

"Make it legal, but regulated," Abrams recommended. "Like tobacco or alcohol." The evidence to support it will emerge gradually, he says. We'll figure out how it works, and who benefits and who doesn't, in much the same way that we've learned about tobacco's ill effects and alcohol's beneficial ones, for instance.

That seems like a rather modest goal for someone who has been at the forefront of the medical marijuana movement for decades. Abrams is convinced of marijuana's benefits—that much is very clear. Yet despite his experience—or rather because of it—he's not optimistic about the possibility of advancing the science to help people. Studies are hard to do, funding is hard to come by, and it will be very hard to get people to listen to the results of those studies.

So, much to my surprise, I find that I'm much more enthusiastic about legalizing medical marijuana than I was a year ago. Not because it always works, because it doesn't always. Nor is it always safe. But more widespread use, with careful safeguards and monitoring and testing, could let us learn a great deal, much faster than we ever could if we rely solely on randomized controlled trials.

That may sound like I'm advocating that we make marijuana available and then figure out whether it works, which would be a backward way of doing science. But that's not what I'm suggesting. We know that marijuana works for some symptoms, like nausea and neuropathic pain. And that should be enough, I think, to justify making it available.

I also think there's enough evidence to justify reclassifying the cannabinoids in marijuana as Schedule II drugs, which include morphine and oxycodone. These are commonly prescribed but are regulated— just as Abrams recommended. And, given all that we know about the benefits of THC and CBD, a reclassification is long overdue. It's no longer fair to say that marijuana deserves a Schedule I classification, reserved for drugs that offer no clinical use. That change will make it easier to do randomized controlled trials, producing more of the evidence we need to use this stuff correctly and safely.

In the meantime, though, why don't we give the public a role in research? Let patients like Rachel and Joseph and Alice try it. Let them see what happens. And then let their experiences guide the design of rigorous trials that reflect the wisdom of the crowd.

That said, crowdsourced science only works if there's a way to make sure that those crowds are well informed and safe. That, in turn, requires much more rigorous medical evaluation than what I experienced in my visit to the first medical marijuana clinic. I shouldn't have been able to lie about my residency to get a letter of recommendation, for instance. And "disturbing feelings" shouldn't have been a qualifying condition for being permitted to fire up a joint.

Anyone thinking about using medical marijuana should seek counseling about its risks. They should also face some restrictions, or at least warnings, if they have a high likelihood of running into trouble. I'm thinking in particular about people with coronary artery disease or a history of schizophrenia, and women who are pregnant. And we've established the risks of driving while high.

There should also be education about potential side effects and dosing, just as there is for any other medication. And there should be enough testing so that users have a pretty good idea of what they're using. Enough of an idea, at least, that they can avoid the hassles of dancing patio furniture and air traffic controllers camped out in their living rooms.

And, finally—although this is probably going to annoy proponents of medical marijuana—there should be some provision for counseling about addiction and monitoring. At a minimum, patients should know that marijuana is addictive. They should also know about the signs of addiction, and when and how to seek help. That would be a good start.

The End of the Road for a Blacksmith and His Boxer

Even if marijuana becomes widely legal and available, that won't happen soon enough for people like Caleb. As far as I know, he never found a reliable source of marijuana that he could afford, or another hospice that would provide it for free. I heard that he left town a month or so after I met him. He loaded Rocky the boxer into his camper and took off for Pueblo, Colorado, in search of marijuana that was more affordable. Or friends with a few buds to spare.

Maybe the crop in the back of his van matured in time for him to harvest it. But maybe not. Last I heard, he was feeling much worse, with more pain that was forcing him to stay in bed almost all day. By late 2014, he'd stopped responding to my e-mails, and even if he is still alive now, as I hope he is, he doesn't have much time left.

It's sad that of all of the patients I've met in the past year, Caleb probably needed marijuana more than most. And yet he couldn't get it. So he left his prescribed drugs in a box in his closet and drove off into the sunset looking for the one drug that he thought could have helped him.

A Brief Marijuana Glossary

Anandamide: One of the body's naturally occurring cannabinoids. Its name is derived from a Sanskrit word (literally "the bliss molecule").

Bhang: Indian preparation of marijuana suspended in ghee (clarified butter).

Bioavailability: A measure of the proportion of a drug that is absorbed. Most cannabinoids ingested by mouth have a bioavailability of 10 to 20 percent. Inhaled, they're 30 to 50 percent.

Bud: The flower of a cannabis plant.

Butane hash oil: Very concentrated cannabinoid-rich oil that is made by using butane to extract cannabinoids from cannabis plants. Other techniques use carbon dioxide or solvents.

Cannabidiol (CBD): One of several dozen naturally occurring cannabinoids. It binds only weakly to CB1 and CB2 receptors in the brain, and does not cause the "high" feeling that THC does.

Cannabidiolic acid: The acidic (and inactive) form of CBD that is present in plants before they're harvested. It's converted to active CBD by drying and heat.

Cannabigerol (CBG): A naturally occurring cannabinoid that is not psychoactive but may slow abnormal cancer growth.

Cannabinoids: A group of molecules that exist in cannabis plants and can also be synthesized in a laboratory.

Cannabis: The genus of the marijuana-producing plant, which includes the species *Cannabis sativa* and *Cannabis indica*. There is disagreement about whether a third group, *Cannabis ruderalis*, is a separate species.

CB1 receptors: Cannabinoid receptors on neurons in the brain and also on cells in the male and female reproductive systems.

CB2 receptors: Cannabinoid receptors on microglial cells in the brain and on immune cells. There are high densities of these receptors where there are concentrations of white blood cells (e.g., in the spleen and gastrointestinal tract).

Concentrates: Substances with very high levels of cannabinoids. These go by names such as oil, wax, shatter, budder, hash, and many others, depending on the consistency of the final product.

Dependence: A term used to describe the state of someone whose use of a drug, like marijuana, is impairing his or her ability to function normally and is causing physical or psychological problems.

Dispensary: A legitimate business that sells marijuana products.

Dravet syndrome: A condition of severe childhood epilepsy caused by a mutation in the SCN1A gene, which is responsible for making channels that allow sodium to flow through a cell membrane.

Dronabinol: A synthetic form of THC, given by mouth, that is available by prescription.

Edibles: Foods that have been infused with marijuana extracts and that contain THC, CBD, and other cannabinoids.

11-OH-tetrahydrocannabinol (11-OH-THC): A metabolite of THC, it is produced in the liver and is at least as psychoactive as THC is. 11-nor-9-carboxy-THC is also a metabolite of THC but is not psychoactive.

First-pass effect: The metabolic "tax" that the liver imposes on a drug taken by mouth, by altering the drug's structure, often making it inactive. (Drugs that are absorbed through the mucosal lining of the mouth or rectum bypass this tax.)

G Protein Receptor 55 (GPR-55): Cannabinoid receptors that have been discovered relatively recently, and that may be one of the ways that CBD reduces childhood seizures. (GPR-18 and GPR-119 are also new receptors, although less well understood.)

Green Dragon: High-proof alcohol that has been infused with marijuana.

Hash: A concentrated form of marijuana, consisting mostly of cannabinoid-rich trichomes from a cannabis plant.

Herbal marijuana: Herbs that may or may not have psychoactive properties, and which are often laced with synthetic cannabinoids.

Indica: Cannabis indica is one species of cannabis that is generally low in THC.

Nabilone: A synthetic cannabinoid developed in the 1970s and still used for the treatment of nausea.

Permeation enhancers: Chemicals like dimethylsulfoxide that help cannabinoid molecules to pass through the skin.

Pistils: Small hairlike fibers found on female cannabis plants that have high cannabinoid concentrations.

Placebo marijuana: Marijuana from which cannabinoids have been removed in the same way that caffeine is removed from coffee beans.

Ruderalis: A form of cannabis that some argue is a separate species. It is generally low in THC and high in CBD, and its flowers are triggered at a certain age rather than by light.

Sativa: Cannabis sativa is a species of cannabis that has relatively high concentrations of THC and has more psychoactive "high" effects than *indica* strains do.

Sativex: A proprietary mixture of THC and CBD that, when dissolved in small amounts of alcohol, can be absorbed through the mucosal lining of the mouth.

Shatter: A form of marijuana concentrate that has the consistency of glass.

Stamen: Part of a flower used to identify male buds; it is low in THC and CBD and thus often culled.

Strain: A variety of a cannabis species. Just as the species of domesticated dogs includes a wide variety of breeds, from Great Danes to dachshunds, one cannabis species (e.g., *sativa* or *indica*) has many strains.

Synthetic cannabinoids: Artificial molecules that share some properties and effects with naturally occurring cannabinoids.

Tetrahydrocannabinol (THC): The most common cannabinoid in marijuana. It is responsible for marijuana's psychoactive effects and the sensation of feeling high.

Tetrahydrocannabinolic acid: The acidic (and inactive) form of THC that is present in plants before they're harvested. It's converted to THC by drying and heat.

Tincture: Cannabinoids that are dissolved in ethanol, typically in very high concentrations.

Trichomes: Very small, hairlike, cannabinoid-rich appendages on cannabis plants.

2-Arachidonoylglycerol: An endocannabinoid, similar to anandamide, that exists in the body and binds to the body's cannabinoid receptors.

Vaporizer: A device that is used to convert to vapor the cannabinoids in marijuana so that they can be inhaled.

Wax: A highly concentrated form of cannabinoids that has a gooey consistency.

The World's Best
(and Simplest)
Brownie Recipe

Steve's recipe for an 8 x 8-inch brownie pan:

½ ounce marijuana	⅓ cup cocoa powder
½ cup vegetable oil	1 cup sugar
¼ teaspoon baking powder	2 eggs
¼ teaspoon salt	1 teaspoon vanilla
½ cup flour	

Grind the marijuana in a coffee grinder or equivalent until it has the consistency of coarse dust. Spread evenly onto a frying pan, preferably nonstick. Use the smallest pan possible and the largest burner available to ensure that the entire surface is evenly heated. Add the vegetable oil. Turn on heat to medium until oil begins to smoke, then turn down to the lowest possible setting. Let the oil/marijuana mixture simmer for at least an hour, stirring frequently. Remove from heat and strain the oil through a coffee filter.

Mix the dry ingredients in one bowl. In a second, larger bowl, mix the marijuana-infused oil and sugar, then add eggs and vanilla. When blended, add the dry ingredients. Pour into a greased 8 x 8-inch pan and bake for 20 minutes at 350 degrees.

Acknowledgments

This book has been a lot of fun to write, for many reasons, not the least of which is that everyone I've met recently seems to have a firm, sometimes strident opinion about medical marijuana. From taxi drivers to college students, they all have something to say. In some ways, that has made my job very easy. Dozens of people have welcomed me into their offices, clinics, laboratories, cars, and mobile homes.

But not everyone was enthusiastic about talking to me. The science of marijuana is still a very new and controversial area, and quite a few people I reached out to declined politely. Others were not so polite. Still others ignored me entirely.

So I'm grateful to those who were willing to put their reputations on the line, especially the researchers who agreed to talk on the record. These include Orrin Devinsky, Teri Franklin, Jonathan Gavrin, Marina Goldman, Steve Lankenau, John Morley, Christine Rabinak, Donald Tashkin, and Barth Wilsey. I'm particularly indebted to Donald Abrams for his efforts to connect me with other researchers. And to Donald and his husband Clint Werner for taking the time to read a version of this manuscript and correct my mistakes.

I'm also grateful to Raphael Mechoulam, who convinced me that the use of medical marijuana is based on real science. He inspired me to take this field of research seriously, but he also cautioned me to be skeptical, just as I would be with any other new drug. So if this book succeeds in balancing optimism and caution, that achievement is thanks in large part to Mechoulam's wise advice.

I also owe a debt to the patients who let me into their lives (and cars) to learn from their experiences. Some used marijuana legally, but many didn't. They've all trusted me to preserve their privacy, and so I can't thank them by name, but they know who they are.

Although patients and researchers may seem to be the stars of this book, the supporting cast is just as important. Thanks to Avinash the marijuana-pushing Nepalese guide and his unnamed hilltop pharmacist. And to Zach Klein, the dragon of Kibbutz Na'an, as well as Justin the hash artisan, Roger the farmer, Jerry the bartender, and Allen the marijuana sommelier. And special thanks to the heavy metal cabdriver in Tel Aviv who taught me how to say "stoned" in between hair-raising lane changes. (It's *mastool*, in case you're interested.) Also thanks to Jan Bezuidenhout, Nathan Pollack, Heather Despres, the pierced receptionist and the strange doctor at the medical marijuana clinic, and Debbie and Larry Gidaley. And, in the animal world, my most special thanks to Buster the cat, Rocky the boxer, Donald Abrams and Clint Werner's dachshunds, Dante and Ruby, and, of course, Sasha the Wonder Dog.

I'm also grateful to the people I work with who keep things running while I'm taking hair-raising taxi rides with Israeli heavy metal drummers and subjecting myself to the ministrations of amateur Nepali pharmacists. Those patient people include Laura Bender, PJ Brennan, Neha Darah, Meredith Dougherty, Joan Doyle, Sue Foster, Sue Kristiniak, Pallavi Kumar, Matt Mendlik, April Nitkin, Nina O'Connor, Anju Ranganathan, and Alana Sagin. I hope the stories I brought home for them were worth it.

On the writing and publishing side, I can always count on Chris Bucci, my agent at Anne McDermid & Associates, for wise advice and an apparently inexhaustible stream of forwarded e-mails about bizarre marijuana use, and (inevitably) stoner jokes. And, once again, I'm grateful to Niki Papadopoulos, Margot Stamas, Kary Perez, and all of the wonderful people at Penguin Random House. They have consistently responded to my marijuana-related writing with an unbridled enthusiasm that has been intensely gratifying (and just a little disturbing).

Notes

Epigraph

1. *The Complete Works of Ralph Waldo Emerson: Miscellanies*, vol. 11 (New York: Houghton Mifflin, 1903–1904), p. 513.

1.
The Blacksmith and the Boxer

1. S. Ryan-Ibarra, M. Induni, and D. Ewing, "Prevalence of medical marijuana use in California, 2012," *Drug and Alcohol Review*, September 26, 2014.

2. B. Freisthler and P. J. Gruenewald, "Examining the relationship between the physical availability of medical marijuana and marijuana use across fifty California cities," *Drug and Alcohol Dependency* 143 (2014): 244–50.

3. M. A. Bloomfield et al., "The link between dopamine function and apathy in cannabis users: An [18F]-DOPA PET imaging study," *Psychopharmacology* 231, no. 11 (2014): 2251–59.

4. *The New York Times*, July 27, 2014, Sunday Review, page 10.

2.
The Girl Who Talked to Cats:
Marijuana's Benefits for the Brain

1. E. B. Russo et al., "Phytochemical and genetic analyses of ancient cannabis from Central Asia," *Journal of Experimental Botany* 59, no. 15 (2008): 4171–82.

2. J. Vargas, "World's oldest marijuana stash totally busted," Discovery News, NBC News, December 3, 2008, http://www.nbcnews.com/id/28034925/ns/

technology_and_science-science/t/worlds-oldest-marijuana-stash-totally-busted/#.VTWcHGZcMt8.

3. Z. Ben-Zvi et al., "6-hydroxy-1-tetrahydrocannabinol synthesis and biological activity," *Science* 174 (1971): 951–52.

4. Clendinning, "Observation on the medicinal properties of Cannabis sativa of India," read May 9 to the British Royal Society of Medicine Medical-Chiurgical Transactions, vol. 26 (1843): 188–210. The following discussion draws on Clendinning's paper, pages 190–92.

5. J. Fiz et al., "Cannabis use in patients with fibromyalgia: Effect on symptoms relief and health-related quality of life," PLoS One [Public Library of Science] (2011); 6(4): e18440. See also M. E. Lynch, J. Young, and A. J. Clark, "A case series of patients using medicinal marihuana for management of chronic pain under the Canadian Marihuana Medical Access Regulations," *Journal of Pain and Symptom Management* 32, no. 5 (2006): 497–501.

6. M. A. Ware et al., "Smoked cannabis for chronic neuropathic pain: A randomized controlled trial," *Canadian Medical Association Journal* 182, no. 14 (2010): E694–701. See also D. R. Blake et al., "Preliminary assessment of the efficacy, tolerability and safety of a cannabis-based medicine (Sativex) in the treatment of pain caused by rheumatoid arthritis," *Rheumatology* 45, no. 1 (Oxford, U.K., 2006): 50–52; D. J. Rog, "Randomized, controlled trial of cannabis-based medicine in central pain in multiple sclerosis," *Neurology* 65, no. 6 (2005): 812–19; and T. J. Nurmikko, "Sativex successfully treats neuropathic pain characterised by allodynia: A randomised, double-blind, placebo-controlled clinical trial," *Pain* 133, nos. 1–3 (2007): 210–20.

7. E. B. Russo, G. W. Guy, and P. J. Robson, "Cannabis, pain, and sleep: Lessons from therapeutic clinical trials of Sativex, a cannabis-based medicine," *Chemistry & Biodiversity* 4, no. 8 (2007): 1729–43.

8. D. A. Gorelick et al., "Around-the-clock oral THC effects on sleep in male chronic daily cannabis smokers," *American Journal on Addictions* 22, no. 22 (2013): 510–14.

9. M. J. Hurley, D. C. Mash, and P. Jenner, "Expression of cannabinoid CB1 receptor mRNA in basal ganglia of normal and parkinsonian human brain," *Journal of Neural Transmission* 110, no. 11 (2003): 1279–88.

10. G. A. Cabral and L. Griffin-Thomas, "Emerging role of the cannabinoid receptor CB2 in immune regulation: Therapeutic prospects for neuroinflammation," *Expert Reviews in Molecular Medicine* 11, no. 1 (2009): e3.

11. B. G. Ramirez et al., "Prevention of Alzheimer's disease pathology by cannabinoids: Neuroprotection mediated by blockade of microglial activation," *Journal of Neuroscience* 25, no. 8 (2005): 1904–13.

12. B. M. Nguyen et al., "Effect of marijuana use on outcomes in traumatic brain injury," *American Surgeon* 80, no. 10 (2014): 979–83.

13. K. Mishima et al., "Cannabidiol prevents cerebral infarction via a serotonergic 5-hydroxytryptamine1A receptor-dependent mechanism," *Stroke* 36, no. 5 (2005): 1077–82.

14. M. P. Castelli et al., "Δ9-tetrahydrocannabinol prevents methamphetamine-induced neurotoxicity." PLoS One (2014) 9: e98079. See also J. Nader et al., "Prior stimulation of the endocannabinoid system prevents methamphetamine-induced dopaminergic neurotoxicity in the striatum through activation of CB2 receptors," *Neuropharmacology* 87 (2014): 214–21.

15. C. J. Morgan et al., "Impact of cannabidiol on the acute memory and psychotomimetic effects of smoked cannabis: Naturalistic study: Naturalistic study [corrected]," *British Journal of Psychiatry* 197, no. 4 (2010): 285–90.

16. M. J. Wright Jr., S. A. Vandewater, and M. A. Taffe, "Cannabidiol attenuates deficits of visuospatial associative memory induced by Δ9 tetrahydrocannabinol," *British Journal of Pharmacology* 170, no. 7 (2013): 1365–73.

17. K. Hayakawa et al., "Cannabidiol potentiates pharmacological effects of Δ9-tetrahydrocannabinol via CB1 receptor-dependent mechanism," *Brain Research* 1188 (2008): 157–64.

18. E. Russo et al., "Agonistic properties of cannabidiol at 5-HT1a receptors," *Neurochemical Research* 30, no. 8 (2005): 1037–43.

19. B. E. Porter and C. Jacobson, "Report of a parent survey of cannabidiol-enriched cannabis use in pediatric treatment-resistant epilepsy," *Epilepsy & Behavior* 29, no. 3 (2013): 574–77.

20. E. A. Carlini, R. Mechoulam, and N. Lander, "Anticonvulsant activity of four oxygenated cannabidiol derivatives," *Research Communications in Chemical Pathology and Pharmacology* 12, no. 1 (1975): 1–15.

21. P. Consroe et al., "Effects of cannabidiol on behavioral seizures caused by convulsant drugs or current in mice," *European Journal of Pharmacology* 83, nos. 3–4 (1982): 293–98.

22. T. D. Hill et al., "Cannabidivarin-rich cannabis extracts are anticonvulsant in mouse and rat via a CB1 receptor-independent mechanism," *British Journal of Pharmacology* 170, no. 3 (2013): 679–92.

23. M. J. Wallace et al., "Assessment of the role of CB1 receptors in cannabinoid anticonvulsant effects," *European Journal of Pharmacology* 428, no. 1 (2001): 51–57.

24. D. Gloss and B. Vickrey, "Cannabinoids for epilepsy," *Cochrane Database of Systematic Reviews* (2012) 6: CD009270.

25. O. Devinsky et al., "Cannabidiol: Pharmacology and potential therapeutic role in epilepsy and other neuropsychiatric disorders," *Epilepsia* 55, no. 6 (2014): 791–802.

26. American Academy of Opthalmology, "American Academy of Ophthalmology reiterates position that marijuana is not proven treatment for glaucoma," White paper, June 24, 2014. http://www.aao.org/newsroom/release/ academy-reiterates-position-that-marijuana-not-proven-glaucoma -treatment.cfm.

27. G. R. Greer, C. S. Grob, and A. L. Halberstadt, "PTSD symptom reports of patients evaluated for the New Mexico medical cannabis program," *Journal of Psychoactive Drugs* 46, no. 1 (2014): 73–77.

28. M. Mashiah, "Medical cannabis as treatment for chronic combat PTSD," presented at the Patients Out of Time Conference, Tucson, Ariz., April 28, 2012.

29. C. A. Rabinak et al., "Cannabinoid facilitation of fear extinction memory recall in humans," *Neuropharmacology* 64 (2013): 396–402.

30. R. K. Das et al., "Cannabidiol enhances consolidation of explicit fear extinction in humans," *Psychopharmacology* 226, no. 4 (2013): 781–92.

31. M. M. Bergamaschi et al., "Cannabidiol reduces the anxiety induced by simulated public speaking in treatment-naive social phobia patients," *Neuropsychopharmacology* 36, no. 6 (2011): 1219–26.

32. J. A. Crippa et al., "Neural basis of anxiolytic effects of cannabidiol (CBD) in generalized social anxiety disorder: A preliminary report," *Journal of Psychopharmacology* 25, no. 1 (2011): 121–30.

3.
The Woman with Knives in Her Neck:
Marijuana's Benefits for the Body

1. B. Wilsey et al., "Low-dose vaporized cannabis significantly improves neuropathic pain," *Journal of Pain* 14, no. 2 (2013): 136–48. See also B. Wilsey et al., "A randomized, placebo-controlled, crossover trial of cannabis cigarettes in neuropathic pain," *Journal of Pain* 9, no. 6 (2008): 506–21; M. E. Lynch and F. Campbell, "Cannabinoids for treatment of chronic non-cancer pain; a systematic review of randomized trials," *British Journal of Clinical Pharmacology* 72, no. 5 (2011): 735–44; and D. I. Abrams et al., "Cannabis in painful HIV-associated sensory neuropathy: A randomized placebo-controlled trial," *Neurology* 68, no. 7 (2007): 515–21.

2. J. P. Zajicek et al., "Multiple sclerosis and extract of cannabis: Results of the MUSEC trial," *Journal of Neurology, Neurosurgery, and Psychiatry* 83, no. 11 (2012): 1125–32.

3. A. Novotna et al., "A randomized, double-blind, placebo-controlled, parallel-group, enriched-design study of nabiximols* (Sativex`), as add-on therapy, in subjects with refractory spasticity caused by multiple sclerosis," *European Journal of Neurology* 18, no. 9 (2011): 1122–31.

4. R. M. Langford et al., "A double-blind, randomized, placebo-controlled, parallel-group study of THC/CBD oromucosal spray in combination with the existing treatment regimen, in the relief of central neuropathic pain in patients with multiple sclerosis," *Journal of Neurology* 260, no. 4 (2013): 984–97. See also D. J. Rog et al., "Randomized, controlled trial of cannabis-based medicine in central pain in multiple sclerosis," *Neurology* 65, no. 6 (2005): 812–19.

5. M. Mecha et al., "Cannabidiol provides long-lasting protection against the deleterious effects of inflammation in a viral model of multiple sclerosis: A role for A2A receptors," *Neurobiology of Disease* 59 (2013): 141–50.

6. B. Zajicek et al., "Effect of dronabinol on progression in progressive multiple sclerosis (CUPID): A randomised, placebo-controlled trial," *Lancet Neurology* 12, no. 9 (2013): 857–65.

7. B. S. Koppel et al., "Systematic review: Efficacy and safety of medical marijuana in selected neurologic disorders. Report of the Guideline Development Subcommittee of the American Academy of Neurology," *Neurology* 82, no. 17 (2014): 1556–63. See also O. Fernández, "Advances in the management of multiple sclerosis spasticity: Recent clinical trials," *European Journal of Neurology* 72, Suppl. 1 (2014): 9–11.

8. B. Pavisian et al., "Effects of cannabis on cognition in patients with MS: A psychometric and MRI study," *Neurology* 82, no. 21 (2014): 1879–87.

9. B. Kraft et al., "Lack of analgesia by oral standardized cannabis extract on acute inflammatory pain and hyperalgesia in volunteers," *Anesthesiology* 109, no. 1 (2008): 101–10.

10. D. I. Abrams et al., "Cannabinoid-opioid interaction in chronic pain," *Clinical Pharmacology and Therapeutics* 90, no. 6 (2011): 844–51.

11. F. C. Machado Rocha et al., "Therapeutic use of *Cannabis sativa* on chemotherapy-induced nausea and vomiting among cancer patients: Systematic review and meta-analysis," *European Journal of Cancer Care* 17, no. 5 (2008): 431–43. See also M. Guzmán, "Cannabinoids: Potential anticancer agents," *Nature Reviews Cancer* 3, no. 10 (2003): 745–55.

12. A. Niiranen and K. Mattson, "A cross-over comparison of nabilone and prochlorperazine for emesis induced by cancer chemotherapy," *American Journal of Clinical Oncology* 8, no. 4 (1985): 336–40. See also L. Lemberger and H. Rowe, "Clinical pharmacology of nabilone, a cannabinol derivative," *Clinical Pharmacology & Therapeutics* 18, no. 6 (1975): 720–26; T. S.

Herman et al., "Nabilone: A potent antiemetic cannabinol with minimal euphoria," *Biomedicine* 27, nos. 9–10 (1977): 331–34.

13. M. Herkenham et al., "Cannabinoid receptor localization in brain," *Neurobiology* 87 (1990): 1932–36.

14. A. H. Söderpalm, A. Schuster, and H. de Wit., "Antiemetic efficacy of smoked marijuana: Subjective and behavioral effects on nausea induced by syrup of ipecac," *Pharmacology, Biochemistry, and Behavior* 69, nos. 3–4 (2001): 343–50.

15. R. W. Foltin, M. W. Fischman, and M. F. Byrne, "Effects of smoked marijuana on food intake and body weight of humans living in a residential laboratory," *Appetite* 11, no. 1 (1988): 1–14.

16. M. Haney et al., "Dronabinol and marijuana in HIV+ marijuana smokers: Acute effects on caloric intake and mood," *Psychopharmacology* 181, no. 1 (2005): 170–78.

17. P. K. Riggs et al., "A pilot study of the effects of cannabis on appetite hormones in HIV-infected adult men," *Brain Research* 1431 (2012): 46–52.

18. E. E. Lutge, A. Gray, and N. Siegfried, "The medical use of cannabis for reducing morbidity and mortality in patients with HIV/AIDS," *Cochrane Database of Systematic Reviews* (2013) 4: CD005175.

19. A. Jatoi et al., "Dronabinol versus megestrol acetate versus combination therapy for cancer-associated anorexia: A North Central Cancer Treatment Group study," *Journal of Clinical Oncology* 20, no. 2 (2002): 567–73. See also F. Strasser et al., "Comparison of orally administered cannabis extract and delta-9-tetrahydrocannabinol in treating patients with cancer-related anorexia-cachexia syndrome: A multicenter, phase III, randomized, double-blind, placebo-controlled clinical trial from the Cannabis-in-Cachexia-Study-Group," *Journal of Clinical Oncology* 24, no. 21 (2006): 3394–400.

20. J. E. Beal et al., "Dronabinol as a treatment for anorexia associated with weight loss in patients with AIDS," *Journal of Pain & Symptom Management* 10, no. 2 (1995): 89–97.

21. "Rick Simpson's hemp-oil medicine," *High Times*, November 13, 2013, http://www.hightimes.com/read/rick-simpsons-hemp-oil-medicine.

22. F. Borrelli et al., "Colon carcinogenesis is inhibited by the TRPM8 antagonist cannabigerol, a Cannabis-derived non-psychotropic cannabinoid," *Carcinogenesis* 3, no. 12 (2014): 2787–97.

23. S. D. McAllister et al., "Pathways mediating the effects of cannabidiol on the reduction of breast cancer cell proliferation, invasion and metastasis," *Breast Cancer Research and Treatment* 129, no. 1 (2011): 37–47.

24. M. Guzmán et al., "A pilot clinical study of Delta9-tetrahydrocannabinol in patients with recurrent glioblastoma multiforme," *British Journal of Cancer* 95, no. 2 (2006): 197–203.

4.
Beer and Brownies

1. U.S. Bureau of Narcotics, *Marihuana: Its Identification*. Washington, D.C.: U.S. Government Printing Office, July 1938.

2. L. Grlić, "Peroxide-sulphuric acid test as an indication of the ripeness and physiological activity of cannabis resin," *Journal of Pharmacy and Pharmacology* 13, no. 1 (1961): 637–38.

3. M. Santos et al., "Effects of *Cannabis sativa* (Marihuana) on the fighting behavior of mice," *Psychopharmacologia* 8, no. 6 (1966): 437–44.

4. S. Valiveti et al., "Transdermal permeation of WIN 55,212-2 and CP 55,940 in human skin in vitro," *International Journal of Pharmaceutics* 278, no. 1 (2004): 173–80.

5. B. N. Nalluri and A. L. Stinchcomb, "Transdermal delivery of cannabidiol," Google Patents, WO 2007001891 A1, 2013.

6. A. L. Stinchcomb et al., "Human skin permeation of Delta8-tetrahydrocannabinol, cannabidiol and cannabinol," *Journal of Pharmacy and Pharmacology* 56, no. 3 (2004): 291–97.

7. M. Lodzki et al., "Cannabidiol-transdermal delivery and anti-inflammatory effect in a murine model," *Journal of Controlled Release* 93, no. 3 (2003): 377–87.

8. W. B. O'Shaughnessy, "On the preparations of the Indian hemp, or gunjah (Cannabis indica): Their effects on the animal system in health, and their utility in the treatment of tetanus and other convulsive diseases," *Provincial Medical Journal* (1843): 363–69. The following quotations are from this report.

9. C. G. Stott et al., "A phase I study to assess the effect of food on the single dose bioavailability of the THC/CBD oromucosal spray," *European Journal of Clinical Pharmacology* 69, no. 4 (2013): 825–34.

5.
Bongs and Budder

1. D. I. Abrams et al., "Vaporization as a smokeless cannabis delivery system: A pilot study," *Clinical Pharmacology & Therapeutics* 82, no. 5 (2007): 572–78.

2. T. P. Freeman et al., "Just say 'know': How do cannabinoid concentrations influence users' estimates of cannabis potency and the amount they roll in joints?" *Addiction* 109, no. 10 (2014): 1686–94.

3. D. I. Abrams et al., "Vaporization as a smokeless cannabis delivery system: A pilot study," *Clinical Pharmacology & Therapeutics* 82, no. 5 (2007): 572–78.

4. D. B. Macleod et al., "Inhaled fentanyl aerosol in healthy volunteers: Pharmacokinetics and pharmacodynamics," *Anesthesia & Analgesia* 115, no. 5 (2012): 1071–77.

5. C. Bullen et al., "Effect of an electronic nicotine delivery device (e cigarette) on desire to smoke and withdrawal, user preferences and nicotine delivery: Randomised cross-over trial," *Tobacco Control* 19, no. 2 (2010): 98–103.

6. A. R. Vansickel et al., "A clinical laboratory model for evaluating the acute effects of electronic 'cigarettes': Nicotine delivery profile and cardiovascular and subjective effects," *Cancer Epidemiology, Biomarkers & Prevention* 19, no. 8 (2010): 1945–53.

7. E. L. Karschner et al., "Implications of plasma Delta9-tetrahydrocannabinol, 11-hydroxy-THC, and 11-nor-9-carboxy-THC concentrations in chronic cannabis smokers," *Journal of Analytical Toxicology* 33, no. 8 (2009): 469–77.

8. P. Mura et al., "THC can be detected in brain while absent in blood," *Journal of Analytical Toxicology* 29, no. 8 (2005): 842–43.

9. N. Gunasekaran et al., "Reintoxication: The release of fat-stored Δ9-tetrahydrocannabinol (THC) into blood is enhanced by food deprivation or ACTH exposure," *British Journal of Pharmacology* 158, no. 5 (2009): 1330–37.

10. A. Wong et al., "Exercise increases plasma THC concentrations in regular cannabis users," *Drug and Alcohol Dependence* 133, no. 2 (2013): 763–67.

11. A. A. Westin et al., "Can Physical Exercise or Food Deprivation Cause Release of Fat-Stored Cannabinoids?" *Basic & Clinical Pharmacology & Toxicology* 115, no. 5 (2014): 467–71.

12. N. Happyana et al., "Analysis of cannabinoids in laser-microdissected trichomes of medicinal Cannabis sativa using LCMS and cryogenic NMR," *Phytochemistry* 83 (2013): 51–59.

6.
Reefer Madness

1. N. Solowij et al., "Cognitive functioning of long-term heavy cannabis users seeking treatment," *Journal of the American Medical Association (JAMA)* 287, no. 9 (2002): 1123–31.

2. A. Batalla et al., "Structural and functional imaging studies in chronic cannabis users: A systematic review of adolescent and adult findings," PLoS One 8, no. 2 (2013): e55821.

3. G. Jager et al., "Long-term effects of frequent cannabis use on working memory and attention: An fMRI study," *Psychopharmacology* 185, no. 3 (2006): 358–68.

4. M. Yucel et al., "Regional brain abnormalities associated with long-term heavy cannabis use," *Archives of General Psychiatry* 65, no. 6 (2008): 694–701.

5. J. Cousijn et al., "Grey matter alterations associated with cannabis use: Results of a VBM study in heavy cannabis users and healthy controls," *Neuroimage* 59, no. 4 (2012): 3845–51. See also J. M. Gilman et al., "Cannabis use is quantitatively associated with nucleus accumbens and amygdala abnormalities in young adult recreational users," *Journal of Neuroscience* 34, no. 16 (2014): 5529–38.

6. T. McQueeny et al., "Gender effects on amygdala morphometry in adolescent marijuana users," *Behavioural Brain Research* 224, no. 1 (2011): 128–34.

7. T. Demirakca et al., "Diminished gray matter in the hippocampus of cannabis users: Possible protective effects of cannabidiol," *Drug and Alcohol Dependence* 114, nos. 2–3 (2011): 242–45.

8. M. Large et al., "Cannabis use and earlier onset of psychosis: A systematic meta-analysis," *Archives of General Psychiatry* 68, no. 6 (2011): 555–61. See also R. Kuepper et al., "Continued cannabis use and risk of incidence and persistence of psychotic symptoms: 10 year follow-up cohort study," *British Medical Journal* 342, no. 7796 (2011): d738; E. Manrique-Garcia et al., "Cannabis, schizophrenia and other non-affective psychoses: 35 years of follow-up of a population-based cohort," *Psychological Medicine* 42, no. 6 (2012): 1321–28; D. Goerke and S. Kumra, "Substance abuse and psychosis," *Child & Adolescent Psychiatry Clinics* 22, no. 4 (2013): 643–54; and G. Bernhardson and L. M. Gunne, "Forty-six cases of psychosis in cannabis abusers," *International Journal of the Addictions* 7, no. 1 (1972): 9–16.

9. W. A. van Gastel et al., "Change in cannabis use in the general population: A longitudinal study on the impact on psychotic experiences," *Schizophrenia Research* 157, nos. 1–3 (2014): 266–70.

10. M. Di Forti et al., "Daily use, especially of high-potency cannabis, drives the earlier onset of psychosis in cannabis users," *Schizophrenia Bulletin* 40, no. 6 (2014): 1590–17.

11. L. Buchy et al., "Impact of substance use on conversion to psychosis in youth at clinical high risk of psychosis," *Schizophrenia Research* 156, nos. 2–3 (2014): 277–80.

12. F. Smit, L. Bolier, and P. Cuijpers, "Cannabis use and the risk of later schizophrenia: A review," *Addiction* 99, no. 4 (2004): 425–30.

13. G. N. Giordano et al., "The association between cannabis abuse and subsequent schizophrenia: A Swedish national co-relative control study," *Psychological Medicine* 45, no. 2 (2014): 407–14.

14. A. C. Proal et al., "A controlled family study of cannabis users with and without psychosis," *Schizophrenia Research* 152, no. 1 (2014): 283–88.

15. P. van der Pol et al., "Mental health differences between frequent cannabis users with and without dependence and the general population," *Addiction* 108, no. 8 (2013): 1459–69.

16. M. Rylander, C. Valdez, and A. M. Nussbaum, "Does the legalization of medical marijuana increase completed suicide?" *American Journal of Drug and Alcohol Abuse* 40, no. 4 (2014): 269–73

17. D. M. Fergusson et al., "Early reactions to cannabis predict later dependence," *Archives of General Psychiatry* 60, no. 10 (2003): 1033–39.

18. W. M. Compton et al., "Prevalence of marijuana use disorders in the United States: 1991–1992 and 2001–2002," *JAMA* 291, no. 17 (2004): 2114–21.

19. J. D. Fraser, "Withdrawal symptoms in cannabis indica addicts," *Lancet* 2 (1949): 748.

20. American Psychiatric Association, "Highlights of Changes from DSM-IV-TR to DSM-V" (PDF), American Psychiatric Association, May 17, 2013: 16.dsm5.org/Documents/changes.

21. D. J. Allsop et al., "Quantifying the clinical significance of cannabis withdrawal," PLoS One 7, no. 9 (2012): e44864.

22. D. Lee et al., "Cannabis withdrawal in chronic, frequent cannabis smokers during sustained abstinence within a closed residential environment," *American Journal on Addictions* 23, no. 3 (2014): 234–42. See also U. Bonnet et al., "Abstinence phenomena of chronic cannabis-addicts prospectively monitored during controlled inpatient detoxification: Cannabis withdrawal syndrome and its correlation with delta-9-tetrahydrocannabinol and -metabolites in serum," *Drug and Alcohol Dependence* 143 (2014): 189–97.

23. D. A. Gorelick et al., "Diagnostic criteria for cannabis withdrawal syndrome," *Drug and Alcohol Dependence* 123, nos. 1–3 (2012): 141–47.

24. M. Loflin and M. Earleywine, "A new method of cannabis ingestion: The dangers of dabs?" *Addictive Behaviors* 39, no. 10 (2014): 1430–33.

25. K. K. Kedzior and L. T. Laeber, "A positive association between anxiety disorders and cannabis use or cannabis use disorders in the general population—a meta-analysis of 31 studies," BMC Psychiatry, BioMed Central Ltd., 2014.

26. R. Secades-Villa et al., "Probability and predictors of the cannabis gateway effect: A national study," *International Journal on Drug Policy* 26, no. 2 (2015): 135–42.

27. M. Li et al., "Marijuana use and motor vehicle crashes," *Epidemiologic Reviews* 34, no. 1 (2012): 65–72.

28. M. Asbridge, J. A. Hayden, and J. L. Cartwright, "Acute cannabis consumption and motor vehicle collision risk: Systematic review of observational studies and meta-analysis," *British Medical Journal* 344, no. 7846 (2012): e536.

29. M. Asbridge et al., "Cycling-related crash risk and the role of cannabis and alcohol: A case-crossover study," *Preventive Medicine* 66 (2014): 80–86.

30. National Highway Traffic and Safety Administration, http://www.nhtsa.gov/people/injury/research/job185drugs/cannabis.htm.

31. D. S. Janowsky et al., "Simulated flying performance after marihuana intoxication," *Aviation, Space, and Environmental Medicine* 47, no. 2 (1976): 124–28. *Aviation, Space, and Environmental Medicine* journal is now published as *Aerospace Medicine and Human Performance*.

32. W. M. Bosker et al., "Medicinal Δ9-tetrahydrocannabinol (dronabinol) impairs on-the-road driving performance of occasional and heavy cannabis users but is not detected in Standard Field Sobriety Tests," *Addiction* 107, no. 10 (2012): 1837–44.

33. L. A. Downey et al., "The effects of cannabis and alcohol on simulated driving: Influences of dose and experience," *Accident Analysis & Prevention* 50, no. 4 (2013): 879–86.

34. J. Bergeron and M. Paquette, "Relationships between frequency of driving under the influence of cannabis, self-reported reckless driving and risk-taking behavior observed in a driving simulator," *Journal of Safety Research* 49 (2014): 19–24.

35. G. Battistella et al., "Weed or wheel! FMRI, behavioural, and toxicological investigations of how cannabis smoking affects skills necessary for driving," *PLoS One* 8, no. 1 (2013): e52545.

36. W. M. Bosker et al., "A placebo-controlled study to assess standardized field sobriety tests performance during alcohol and cannabis intoxication in heavy cannabis users and accuracy of point of collection testing devices for detecting THC in oral fluid," *Psychopharmacology* 223, no. 4 (2012): 439–46.

7.

Bodily Harm

1. D. P. Tashkin, "Effects of marijuana smoking on the lung," *Annals of the American Thoracic Society* 10, no. 3 (2013): 239–47.

2. D. P. Tashkin et al., "Heavy habitual marijuana smoking does not cause an accelerated decline in FEV1 with age," *American Journal of Respiratory and Critical Care Medicine* 155, no. 1 (1997): 141–48.

3. R. J. Hancox et al., "Effects of cannabis on lung function: A population-based cohort study," *European Respiratory Journal* 35, no. 1 (2010): 42–47.

4. M. Pletcher et al., "Association between marijuana exposure and pulmonary function over 20 years." *JAMA* 307, no. 2 (2012): 173–81.

5. M. H. Lee and R. J. Hancox, "Effects of smoking cannabis on lung function," *Expert Reviews in Respiratory Medicine* 5, no. 4 (2011): 537–46.

6. J. M. Tetrault et al., "Effects of marijuana smoking on pulmonary function and respiratory complications: A systematic review," *Archives of Internal Medicine* 167, no. 3 (2007): 221–28.

7. S. J. Williams, J. P. Hartley, and J. D. Graham, "Bronchodilator effect of delta1-tetrahydrocannabinol administered by aerosol of asthmatic patients," *Thorax* 31, no. 6 (1976): 720–23.

8. M. Hashibe et al., "Epidemiologic review of marijuana use and cancer risk," *Alcohol* 35, no. 3 (2005): 265–75.

9. L. R. Zhang et al., "Cannabis smoking and lung cancer risk: Pooled analysis in the International Lung Cancer Consortium," *International Journal of Cancer* 136, no. 4 (2014): 894–903.

10. R. C. Callaghan, P. Allebeck, and A. Sidorchuk, "Marijuana use and risk of lung cancer: A 40-year cohort study," *Cancer Causes and Control* 24, no. 10 (2013): 1811–20.

11. N. T. Van Dam and M. Earleywine, "Pulmonary function in cannabis users: Support for a clinical trial of the vaporizer," *International Journal on Drug Policy* 21, no. 6 (2010): 511–13.

12. C. F. Schaefer, C. G. Gunn, and K. M. Dubowski, "Letter: Marihuana dosage control through heart rate," *New England Journal of Medicine* 293, no. 2 (1975): 101.

13. M. A. Mittleman et al., Triggering myocardial infarction by marijuana, *Circulation* (2001) 103: 2805–9.

14. E. Deusch et al., "The procoagulatory effects of delta-9-tetrahydrocannabinol in human platelets," *Anesthesia & Analgesia* 99, no. 4 (2004): 1127–30, table of contents.

15. K. J. Mukamal et al., "An exploratory prospective study of marijuana 15 and mortality following acute myocardial infarction," *American Heart Journal* 155, no. 3 (2008): 465–70.

16. L. Frost et al., "Marijuana use and long-term mortality among survivors of acute myocardial infarction," *American Heart Journal* 165, no. 2 (2013): 170–75.

17. V. Wolff et al., "Cannabis use, ischemic stroke, and multifocal intracranial vasoconstriction: A prospective study in 48 consecutive young patients,"

Stroke 42, no. 6 (2011): 1778–80. See also N. N. Singh et al., "Cannabis-related stroke: Case series and review of literature," *Journal of Stroke and Cerebrovascular Diseases* 21, no. 7 (2012): 555–60.

18. P. A. Barber et al., "Cannabis, ischemic stroke, and transient ischemic attack: A case-control study," *Stroke* 44, no. 8 (2013): 2327–29.

19. M. Earleywine, "Cannabis-induced Koro in Americans," *Addiction* 96, no. 11 (2001): 1663–66.

20. N. D. Volkow et al., "Adverse health effects of marijuana use," *New England Journal of Medicine* 371, no. 9 (2014): 878.

21. S. E. Nicolson et al., "Cannabinoid hyperemesis syndrome: A case series and review of previous reports," *Psychosomatics* 53, no. 3 (2012): 212–19. See also D. A. Simonetto et al., "Cannabinoid hyperemesis: A case series of 98 patients," *Mayo Clinic Proceedings* 87, no. 2 (2012): 114–19.

22. M. Vallée et al., "Pregnenolone can protect the brain from cannabis intoxication," *Science* 343, no. 6166 (2014): 94–98.

23. M. W. Varner et al., "Association between stillbirth and illicit drug use and smoking during pregnancy," *Obstetrics & Gynecology* 123, no. 1 (2014): 113–25.

24. A. Desai, K. Mark, and M. Terplan, "Marijuana use and pregnancy: Prevalence, associated behaviors, and birth outcomes," *Obstetrics & Gynecology* 123, Suppl. 1 (2014): 46S.

25. J. J. Janisse et al., "Alcohol, tobacco, cocaine, and marijuana use: Relative contributions to preterm delivery and fetal growth restriction," *Substance Abuse* 35, no. 1 (2014): 60–67.

26. D. A. Kosior et al., "Paroxysmal atrial fibrillation in a young female patient following marijuana intoxication—a case report of possible association," *Medical Science Monitor* 6, no. 2 (2000): 386–89.

27. A. C. Lindsay et al., "Cannabis as a precipitant of cardiovascular emergencies," *International Journal of Cardiology* 104, no. 2 (2005): 230–32.

28. A. C. Desbois and P. Cacoub, "Cannabis-associated arterial disease," *Annals of Vascular Surgery* 27, no. 7 (2013): 996–1005. See also H. J. Schneider, S. Jha, and K. G. Burnand, "Progressive arteritis associated with cannabis use," *European Journal of Vascular and Endovascular Surgery* 18, no. 4 (1999): 366–67; and M. Halpern and B. P. Citron, "Necrotizing angiitis associated with drug abuse," *American Journal of Roentgenology, Radium Therapy, and Nuclear Medicine* 111, no. 4 (1971): 663–71. Now published as *American Journal of Roentgenology*.

29. C. E. Rodríguez-Castro et al., "Recurrent myopericarditis as a complication of marijuana use," *American Journal of Case Reports* 15 (2014): 60–62.

30. F. Corvi et al., "Central retinal vein occlusion in a young patient following cannabis smoke inhalation," *European Journal of Ophthalmology* 24, no. 3 (2014): 437–40.

31. B. Skovrlj et al., "Curvularia abscess of the brainstem," *World Neurosurgery* 82, nos. 1–2 (2014): 241.

32. Menahem S., Cardiac asystole following cannabis (marijuana) usage—additional mechanism for sudden death? *Forensic Science International* (2013) 233: e3–5.

33. Y. L. Hurd et al., "Marijuana impairs growth in mid-gestation fetuses," *Neurotoxicology and Teratology* 27, no. 2 (2005): 221–29.

34. R. C. Kolodny et al., "Depression of plasma testosterone levels after chronic intensive marihuana use," *New England Journal of Medicine* 290, no. 16 (1974): 872–74.

35. J. Harmon and M. A. Aliapoulios, "Gynecomastia in marihuana users," *New England Journal of Medicine* 287, no. 18 (1972): 936.

36. H. Fatma et al., "Cannabis: A rare cause of acute pancreatitis," *Clinics and Research in Hepatology and Gastroenterology* 37, no. 1 (2013): e24–25.

37 B. E. Juel-Jensen, "Cannabis and recurrent herpes simplex," *British Medical Journal* 4, no. 4 (1972): 296.

38. National Poison Data System, "Marijuana human exposure data, 2000–2010," available at aapcc.org.

39. A. H. Scheel et al., "Talcum induced pneumoconiosis following inhalation of adulterated marijuana, a case report," *Diagnostic Pathology* 7, no. 1 (2012): 26.

8.
Caveat Emptor

1. C. Reinarman et al., "Who are medical marijuana patients? Population characteristics from nine California assessment clinics," *Journal of Psychoactive Drugs* 43, no. 2 (2011): 128–35.

2. California Compassionate Use Act, available at cdph.ca.gov/programs/mmp/pages/compassionateuseact.aspx.

9.
The Future of Medical Marijuana

1. E. di Tomaso, M. Beltramo, and D. Piomelli, "Brain cannabinoids in chocolate," *Nature* 382, no. 6593 (1996): 677–78.

2. W. A. Devane et al., "Isolation and structure of a brain constituent that binds to the cannabinoid receptor," *Science* 258, no. 5090 (1992): 1946–49.

3. J. McPartland et al., "Cannabinoid receptors are absent in insects," *Journal of Comparative Neurology* 436, no. 4 (2001): 423–29.

4. A. T. Lu et al., "Association of the cannabinoid receptor gene (CNR1) with ADHD and post-traumatic stress disorder," *American Journal of Medical Genetics B: Neuropsychiatric Genetics* 147, no. 8 (2008): 1488–89.

5. E. S. Onaivi., "Neuropsychobiological evidence for the functional presence and expression of cannabinoid CB2 receptors in the brain," *Neuropsychobiology* 54, no. 4 (2006): 231–46.

6. D. Jesudason and G. Wittert., "Endocannabinoid system in food intake and metabolic regulation," *Current Opinion in Lipidology* 19, no. 4 (2008): 344–48.

7. M. Karsak et al., "Cannabinoid receptor type 2 gene is associated with human osteoporosis," *Human Molecular Genetics* 14, no. 22 (2005): 3389–96.

8. L. K. Miller and L. A. Devi, "The highs and lows of cannabinoid receptor expression in disease: Mechanisms and their therapeutic implications," *Pharmacological Reviews* 63, no. 3 (2011): 461–70.

9. L. Lemberger and H. Rowe, "Clinical pharmacology of nabilone, a cannabinol derivative," *Clinical Pharmacology & Therapeutics* 18, no. 6 (1975): 720–26. See also L. Lemberger, "Nabilone: A Synthetic Cannabinoid of Medicinal Utility," in *Marihuana and Medicine*, ed. G. Nahas et al. (Totowa, N.J.: Humana Press, 1999).

10. A. Niiranen and K. Mattson, "Antiemetic efficacy of nabilone and dexamethasone: A randomized study of patients with lung cancer receiving chemotherapy," *American Journal of Clinical Oncology* 10, no. 4 (1987): 325–29. See also A. Niiranen and K. Mattson, "A cross-over comparison of nabilone and prochlorperazine for emesis induced by cancer chemotherapy," *American Journal of Clinical Oncology* 8, no. 4 (1985): 336–40.

11. J. A. Lile, T. H. Kelly, and L. R. Hays, "Substitution profile of the cannabinoid agonist nabilone in human subjects discriminating 9-tetrahydrocannabinol," *Clinical Neuropharmacology* 33, no. 5 (2010): 235–42.

12. A. Rael, "Nicholas Colbert died after smoking synthetic marijuana, now his mother is suing," *Huffington Post*, September 23, 2013. http://wwwZ.huffingtonpost.com/2013/09/23/nicholas-colbert-syntheti_n_3977073.html.

13. J. Steffen, "Mother sues convenience store that sold her son synthetic marijuana," *Denver Post*, September 23, 2013. http://www.denverpost.com/breakingnews/ci_24157901/mother-sues-convenience-store-that-sold-her-son.

14. C. Burnett, "Alleged synthetic pot distributor sued in teen's death," *Atlanta Journal-Constitution,* August 28, 2012, http://www.ajc.com/news/news/crime-law/alleged-synthetic-pot-distributor-sued-in-teens-de/nRMgW.

15. M. J. Freeman et al., "Ischemic stroke after use of the synthetic marijuana 'spice,'" *Neurology* 81, no. 24 (2013): 2090–93.

16. S. Alhadi et al., "High times, low sats: Diffuse pulmonary infiltrates associated with chronic synthetic cannabinoid use," *Journal of Medical Toxicology* 9, no. 2 (2013): 199–206.

17. M. Hermanns-Clausen et al., "Acute toxicity due to the confirmed consumption of synthetic cannabinoids: Clinical and laboratory findings," *Addiction* 108, no. 3 (2013): 534–44.

18. J. Rose, "The Unlikely Clemson Chemist Behind Synthetic Marijuana" (Charlotte, N.C.): WFAE.org. http://wfae.org/post/unlikely-clemson-chemist-behind-synthetic-marijuana.

19. A. M. Malfait et al., "The nonpsychoactive cannabis constituent cannabidiol is an oral anti-arthritic therapeutic in murine collagen-induced arthritis," *Proceedings of the National Academy of Sciences of the United States of America* 97, no. 17 (2000): 9561–66.

20. L. Keen, D. Pereira, and W. Latimer, "Self-reported lifetime marijuana use and interleukin-6 levels in middle-aged African Americans," *Drug and Alcohol Dependence* 140 (2014): 156–60.

10.
A Long Strange Trip

1. I. Lotan et al., "Cannabis (medical marijuana) treatment for motor and non-motor symptoms of Parkinson disease: An open-label observational study," *Clinical Neuropharmacology* 37, no. 2 (2014): 41–44.

2. M. H. Chagas et al., "Effects of cannabidiol in the treatment of patients with Parkinson's disease: An exploratory double-blind trial," *Journal of Psychopharmacology* 28, no. 11 (2014): 1088–92.

Index